UNTIL T
ARE F

Angela Phillips is a freelance journalist. She is the author of *Your Body, Your Baby, Your Life* (also published by Pandora) and the UK co-editor of *Our Bodies, Ourselves* and the *New Our Bodies, Ourselves*. She lives in London with her two children.

UNTIL THEY ARE FIVE

A PARENTS' GUIDE

ANGELA PHILLIPS

Illustrations by Ros Asquith

PANDORA

London Sydney Wellington

First published by Pandora Press, an imprint of the Trade Division of Unwin Hyman Limited in 1989.

Pandora Press
Unwin Hyman Limited
15/17 Broadwick Street
London W1V 1FP

Unwin Hyman Inc
8 Winchester Place, Winchester, MA 01890, USA

Allen & Unwin Australia Pty Ltd
PO Box 764, 8 Napier Street, North Sydney, NSW 2060, Australia

Allen & Unwin New Zealand Pty Ltd with the Port Nicholson Press
Compusales Building, 75 Ghuznee Street, Wellington, New Zealand

Set in Linotron Century by Input Typesetting Ltd, London

British Library Cataloguing in Publication Data
  Philips, Angela
  Until they are five.
  1. Children, to 5 years. Home care
  I. Title
  649′.122

ISBN 0–04–440361–5

To my children
with all my love

CONTENTS

INTRODUCTION

This book is not the work of an 'expert', though some of them have helped in its creation. Rather, it is an attempt to share the thoughts and solutions of parents who have 'been there'. Many of the parents and children on these pages are my friends (though I have changed all their names). Among them are the people who have helped me to cope with the difficult moments and shared the happy ones. Their wit and wisdom has added to my pleasure in being a parent and I thank them all for it. I hope that it will add to your pleasure too.

I have not attempted to provide recipes for successful parenting. A child-care book which provides instructions is of little help to anyone. Our children are not made to formula. What we all need is support, information, and the time and space to make our own decisions. I offer you this book as a contribution to the decisions which you will have to make for yourself, adding only the thought that the best decisions are always the ones which make the most people happy – and that includes us.

In acknowledging the help I have been given on this book I would need to mention most of the parents and children I know as well as many that I do not know. I have decided not to name names because it would make it too easy to identify many of the incidents and children described. I do not believe that any children (my own included) would benefit from having their early years served up as an example to others. May I say to all who helped – thank you. I appreciate it.

Other people gave their time to read my manuscripts and advise me: Kiran Shukla, Dr Anne Kilby, Dr Anne Evans and Eva Lloyd, have all discussed aspects of the material or commented on the finished text. Their advice has been invaluable. I have also turned to other authors and their work has helped me too. These include Anne Oakley, Sue Sharpe, Sheila Kitzinger, Barbara Tizard, Bruno Bettleheim and Rudolph Schaffer. Above all I have been helped, advised, sustained and supported by Linda Phillips, child-minder, crèche organiser, and friend, who has given loving care to my children and so many others.

Chapter 1

BECOMING PARENTS

CHANGING PERSPECTIVES

The time around a birth can feel like a magic island. You and your new child are held in a bubble while friends and relations visit, beaming, with flowers and presents. But it isn't all roses. Having a baby changes everything: our perspective, our sense of time, our relationships. It is the ultimate rite of passage. For the first time in our lives we find ourselves putting someone else's needs first. Not on an occasional basis, like giving an old lady a seat on the bus, but all the time.

'It gradually dawns on you that it's for keeps. For the rest of your life there will be a part of your mind which is reserved for someone else.'

In my experience, which is shared by most of the people I have known, parenthood has been a deeply rewarding experience. The situation and conditions in which we have our children can make life hard, but however much we might rail about the lack of assistance given in our hard-hearted, non-childcentred society, our children are the reward for our efforts, not the punishment for our sins. As one father said to me:

'I just think it's awful that anyone could look back and regret having their child. I look at Mary when I put her to bed and I know I could never love anyone like that. She is irreplaceable.'

Perhaps the most beautiful description of parent love was written by Sara Maitland in *Why Children?* (The Women's Press, 1980):

'I find my daughter movingly, passionately beautiful: when I see her running naked, or coiled sleeping. I feel something which is not (I hope) lust, but alarmingly akin to it – a physical delight and recognition and excitement; and a desire to elicit from her a similar response. And I like her: for her energy and tenderness and sturdy independence; for her wit and intelligence and her passionate sense of her own selfhood.'

Of course there are people who have regrets. Perhaps they fell into parenthood by accident at a time in their lives when they were totally unprepared to make the necessary adjustments, and found themselves sinking under the weight of responsibility.

Though I have rarely heard a mother expressing regret about having children, I have occasionally heard fathers confessing that 'It was a big mistake. I should never have been a father.' Perhaps they are men who feel supplanted by their children and are unable to shift from being the child of their partner to being her equal. Many other fathers feel momentary panic at the enormity of what they have taken on. As Graham observed:

> 'I feared getting totally domesticated, and I feared liking it. I think the feeling was to do with a fanciful idea of male independence. Men are always afraid of missing out on something.'

Men may find it particularly hard to find release for their feelings of fear and guilt, because there is no real tradition of post-childbirth support for them. Often their male friends melt away, leaving them stranded and alone as their partners are welcomed into the sisterhood of mothers.

It is perhaps time that men thought harder about the rôle they could play in supporting each other at this time – not the beer-swilling, back-slapping and commiserating of the traditional male celebration of birth, but real support, an opportunity to talk about feelings with others who have been through this transfiguring experience.

Postnatal depression

Though mothers are more likely to be supported as they enter parenthood, they also face bigger changes in their lives. They are more likely to be leaving the world of work for the first time and they are usually taking on most of the work of childcare and most of the responsibility for their child's welfare. For a significant number of women, fear, and feelings of inadequacy, may become overwhelming. This young single mother was interviewed by Sue Sharpe in *Falling for Love* (Virago, 1987):

> 'I had a terrible postnatal depression. I used to sit and cry. Up until she was about four months old. If anybody said anything to upset me I just burst out crying. That wasn't like me. At the slightest mention of her father's name I got upset. I think if Mum hadn't been there I would have done something to her.'

Postnatal depression can hit anyone: married or single, young or older. It is as likely to hit someone who has been longing for a baby as a young single woman who has become a mother by accident. This depression is partly physical (there is an enormous change in hormone levels after childbirth), but it may be connected to a number of other feelings: the sense of being out of control of your life, the extreme fatigue which often accompanies early

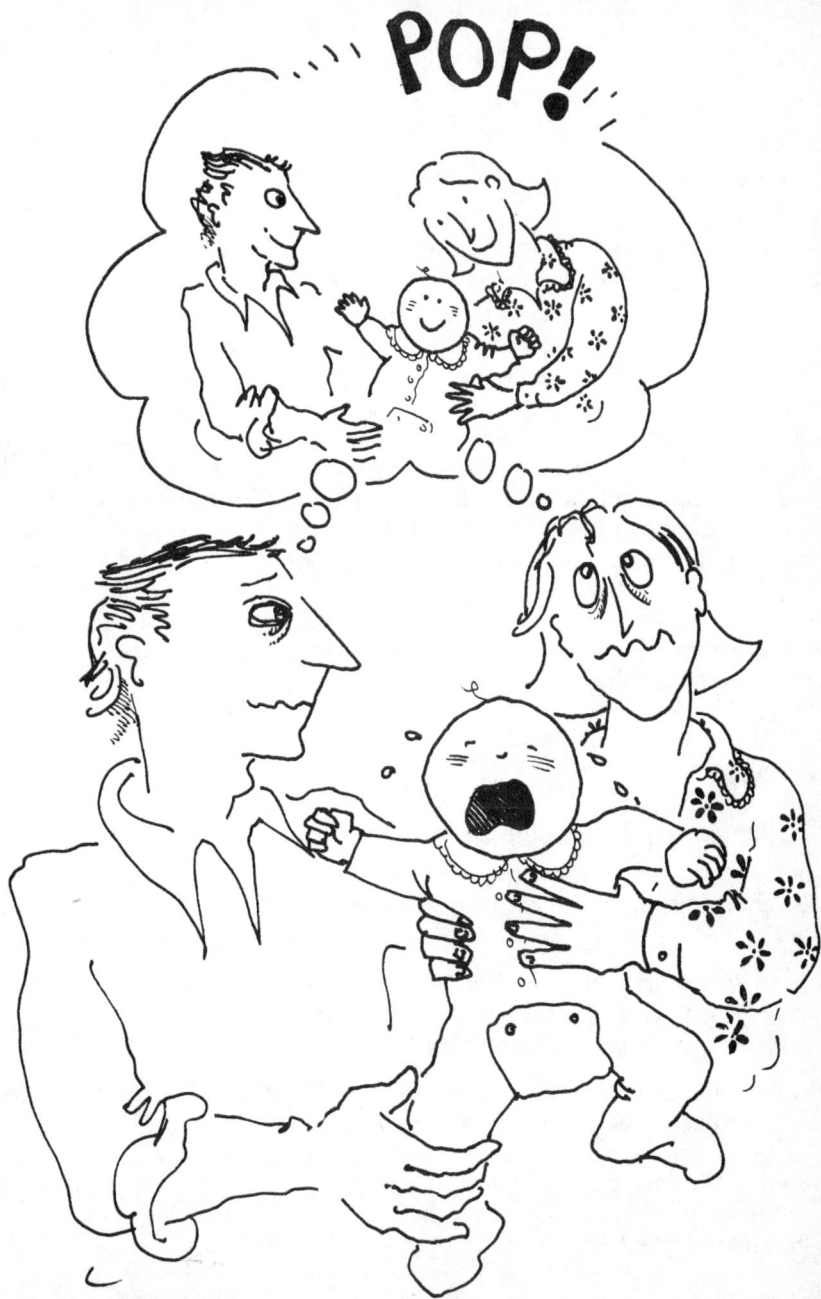

parenthood, and loneliness which can be as bad within a relationship as for a lone parent. Said one father interviewed in an EOC study:

'What I noticed, after the first two she had depression really bad but this time since I've been home she's been great – I think it's directly due to my being home. I've been waiting for the crunch to come but this time she's been really great. I can't see any other reason other than me being here to explain it.'

New mothers shouldn't be alone. It's a sad indictment of our culture that so many women enter this vital and exciting new phase of life without any consistent, caring support. Clinics and health visitors are no substitute for an experienced older relation to help you make this transition. It's amazing, in the circumstances, that the sheer joy of having a baby is a potent enough sensation to carry most of us through these early days of fumbling, experimenting and feeling our way.

If joy is the last word that you would apply to your experience of motherhood, if you find that you are dragging yourself through the day, weeping and unable to cope, you may need help. This is not the way that motherhood should be and it needn't be this way for you. Organisations which provide postnatal support for mothers are listed under 'Help' at the back of this book. If you feel that it is too hard even to make a phonecall, perhaps you need help from your doctor first. Don't feel ashamed to ask for it. Society owes you all the support it can give to ensure that you do not miss out on what should be one of the most positive experiences in your life.

ADJUSTING TO CHILD TIME

The demands of a child do not come in tidy blocks, with tea breaks, like a job. They swing up and down through a twenty-four hour cycle. One mother said as she contemplated returning to work after ten years and three children:

'It's a different kind of time. You are always occupied but everything is broken up in little fragments. The thought of facing a whole day of uninterrupted time is frightening.'

If you are going out to work as well as caring for a child you will have to cope with swinging between two different kinds of time and two different kinds of pace on a daily basis. At work each task can be taken on and completed. At home you are usually juggling several things at once and yet you need to drop your speed down to baby pace. It isn't always easy to make the adjustment, in either direction.

'Once I had a baby, union meetings suddenly seemed different. Where

once I had enjoyed the wrangles and digressions I suddenly found myself impatient. Each new meaningless amendment was time away from my baby. I became one of those people who complains about sloppy chairing.'

Whether you are going out to work and then coming home to care for children, or staying home with them full time, one of the biggest difficulties is simply finding the time and space to think. If you have fallen into parenthood without thinking very hard about it you may find changes taking place in your life which you have not had time to consider. Even when a pregnancy is planned you may feel overwhelmed by the changes. The roundabout is in motion and it's too late to get off.

'When you get married and you've got no kids you can just go and sit in your bedroom and make yourself all nice, but with a kid you don't get time to do nothing, you don't even get a bath. You don't get a chance to just sit down and read a book, they are always there.' (Falling for Love, ibid)

Many mothers report that for months after their babies are born they stop looking in mirrors, may quite literally forget what clothes they are wearing and, more important, stop eating properly. It's the baby's health that you are focussing on, but remind yourself that the baby is dependent on you. Finding time to put yourself first may feel impossible but it could make all the difference between coping with the ups and downs and going under.

Suzie's husband left her before her daughter was a year old. She found herself coping with loss, grief and anger on top of what she now realises was postnatal depression. Part of finding the way out was putting herself first:

'We were living on Social Security and Ray hardly ever gave us money (though he was meant to). I used to spend £5 per week on me. I would go to a sauna, get my hair cut, one week I thought, "here goes this week's" and I got my ears pierced.'

For couples the biggest difficulty may well be finding time to be together and talk about your life. It's so easy to slip into seeing your partner as 'just the other babysitter'. But at a time of profound change no partnership can survive without space for discussion and negotiation. Says Graham:

'Fortunately we have never gone through the thing of never having time to talk to each other. Mary's work meant that she had to be away for at least two days of the week from morning until late evening. It always seemed natural for her to spend time away from Gemma. When we are at home Gemma has lots of attention but she knows that her parents have another life.'

RENEGOTIATING RELATIONSHIPS

Paradoxically, for those of us entering parenthood alone, the adjustment to parenthood may be easier (though the work is usually harder). At least you are only having to adjust your life in one direction. Says Marcelle:

'It works for you and against you. In the first three years single parenthood has advantages. All the attention that could have been devoted to a lover went to her. After that time I felt that she was wondering "why isn't my mother loved?".'

For those of us in partnerships the adjustment can be complex. Not only do you both need to take on board the needs of a new human being but you also have to adjust to the changes in each other. You have to negotiate a new relationship between you as well as initiating a relationship with your child. A quote from *Our Bodies Ourselves* (ed. Phillips and Rakusen) sums it up for me:

'When I think back on it, adding a baby was like sending our relationship through a wringer and planting a garden smack in it's middle – both at once.'

Ann Oakley, in her book *From Here to Maternity* (Pelican, 1981), discovered that:

'The emotional relationship between mother and father seems to improve during pregnancy to a peak just after birth, and then to deteriorate. Birth, a joint achievement, unites husband and wife; the baby, a maternal activity, divides them.'

As her book also points out, it is often the difference in the nature of their occupations which drives a wedge between partners. The partner who goes out returns in the evening with energy and anticipation. The partner at home has been working to a very different rhythm. It doesn't matter whether the stay-at-home partner is a man or a woman.

'I know Lawrence feels a bit left out. Because I'm tired. I used to be an awfully happy, jolly person and I've just been so tired. Lawrence comes in and I flake. I don't get angry. I just get cross. I'm crotchety and I feel emotionally drained. Lawrence feels he's somehow failed me and I feel likewise – that I am not making him happy.'

Where the stay-at-home partner is the man the rift may become even more complicated. While many women would be delighted if their partner came home and 'took over' domestically, for a father who has been at home with the children this assumption of the domestic role can feel like a reproach. A father interviewed in the same book said:

*'Jo's got a habit of coming home and working her arse off – it could
be stitching up those curtains, it could be cleaning bottles, it could
be emptying the nappy bucket. I resent it because really I feel I should
be doing it. And that sort of builds up inside me and so I can't just
bottle it all up and I just turn around and say get out of the fucking
way.'*

A woman who has dropped out of paid work to care for children may well
feel tired, frustrated and angry. She may feel a loss of identity but she
doesn't feel less of a woman. A man who stays home with children may
suffer the same tiredness and frustration much of the time but he is also in
danger of suffering the loss of his identity as a man. Our society doesn't
have a place for male carers. A man who takes on this rôle is often looked
on with suspicion both by other men and by other women. As one lone father
put it: 'If you try to chat to some other bloke's wife the neighbours start
talking.' Another father with major charge of his children felt that women
could only accept him if they 'de-sexualised him'. This made him uneasy
because it threatened his already shaken sexual identity still further.

Parents reaching out across the gap created by their rapidly changing
lives need a high degree of empathy and understanding if they are to reshape
their relationship in a way which satisfies both of them and accommodates
the needs of their children too. Couples who have relied on sex as a way of
settling differences and comforting one another may find it particularly
difficult to make contact.

*'I just lost interest completely. My baby took up all my need for skin
contact. My partner's attentions seemed rough and intrusive and sex
itself seemed somehow ludicrous. It wasn't physical contact I wanted,
it was emotional contact. He seemed to have no idea how much I needed
to feel his tenderness, to feel that he was actually interested in me and
what I was doing. He would work all evening and then want to fuck. I
would feel absolutely enraged and used.'*

Loss of sexual interest is extremely common in the months after a baby is
born. To start with many women feel pain from trauma and stitches which
can take weeks to heal. On top of that comes the fatigue of the early weeks
compounded by a daily routine which has slowed down to baby pace. Come
evening, many child-carers can think of nothing more pleasant than sleep.
This is not a phase which will last for ever. Sexual interest does return
provided that both partners can find other ways to reach out to one another
and give each other love and comfort in the meantime.

Parents who have a genuine understanding of each other's lives have a
far greater chance of negotiating these early changes. When both parents
have experienced the care of children at first hand they understand what
sort of an occupation it is and they are more likely to understand why the

baby's needs must, for a time at least, occupy centre stage. Graham and Mary have had a relatively easy transition into parenthood, which Graham puts down to the fact that he had plenty of time to get to know his baby:

> *'I think it is hard for men who have little to do with their children from early on. They cannot understand how the mother-child relationship has built up and they feel cut out. I was lucky. I got six months off when she was born. If I had only had a couple of weeks it wouldn't have been the same. In fact it's panned out just as Mary said it would. Not as a dependency, a loss, but as a new opportunity.'*

While it may be hard for the partner who feels left out, it can be a great deal harder for the parent who has to cope with a partner who continues to make demands rather than sharing responsibility. Sheila Kitzinger, in her book *The Crying Baby* (Viking, 1989), quotes many instances of men who continue to expect their wives to wait on them hand and foot in spite of the fact that they are clearly already finding it hard to cope with the demands of a small infant:

> *'He expected everything to go on as if nothing had happened. He still expected cooking and household chores to be done as normal.'*

As Kitzinger says: 'For a woman it is as though she has two babies in the house. One is the new baby, the other is the husband. Because the husband is bigger and more powerful he is much the more threatening of the two.'

SHARING PARENTING

In partnerships where baby care is genuinely divided, both partners have the advantage of retaining their identity as people as well as parents. At the same time the care of the children becomes a shared territory, their growing up something to take equal pleasure from, their bad nights a problem to be solved together. Their achievements become a source of shared pride. Says one father:

> *'I was amazed by how quickly I could identify him as a companion rather than just a responsibility and by how he awakened in me an ability to express affection which I had bottled up. With him it just came out so easily.'*

However, shared parenting is far from being the norm even among couples where both parents work. One mother I spoke to who has worked outside the home for most of her child's life, said of her partner: 'I was made to feel guilty every time I walked out of the house and left them together.' As one slightly jaded women's rights officer put it: 'Men may dote, but they don't do.' For a mother who is doing all the work of child care, even a good relationship between father and children can become a source of tension. 'He gets all the fun, I do all the work.'

For Kath, sharing parenting with her lesbian partner who is the biological mother of their child has come easily, but getting recognition from others for her rôle is harder:

'I have as many sleepless nights, I wash as many nappies. I take as much of the responsibility as Judy does. A lot of childless lesbians just don't know what child care is about. I guess that's why heterosexual mothers find it easier to accept us. A lot of them are jealous. To them the idea of two women bringing up a child is wonderful. It's totally clear to them.' (Getting Pregnant Our Way – WHIC)

Sharing is not something that can be imposed by one partner on the other. It must, by definition, be voluntary, and considered. A partner who 'helps when asked' is not sharing – he is leaving the entire onus of organisation on his partner. And work done as a favour has to be 'paid for'. Mothers often complain that they have to 'repay' every bit of 'help' offered tenfold. Yet how often does the man who 'helps' thank his partner for her contribution? Usually he takes it for granted. As a friend quipped: 'Shared parenting depends on how the old man feels: that just about sums it up.'

In partnerships where child care is genuinely shared, even at times when the relationship between the partners is strained, they can communicate effectively about the needs of their children. These partnerships offer their children a high degree of love and security without compromising the needs of the parents for lives of their own. They are worth working at. One father writes:

'For me, with all its difficulties, child care is the best thing in life. It gives me indescribable pleasure and it is profoundly educative. I have learned more about myself over the past few years than I ever did before.'

In the early years there is nearly always some division of labour between parents. I know couples who have taken turns working part time to ensure that the children always have a parent around for part of the day. A more common pattern is for women to work shorter hours than their partners (this nearly always ends up with the mother doing all the child care *and* bringing in more than her fair share of income). Some couples agree that one of them will stay at home while the other works full time, and in some cases both work full time. Whatever the pattern, parenting can still be shared, but that sharing can only work well if partners have a joint view of what their contribution should be.

GETTING SUPPORT

However you choose to divide the jobs of parenting, you will inevitably spend long periods of time alone with your children. There will also be times when you feel the need for support from someone who is not too close to see things in perspective and you will want people to talk to about your experiences.

The doting parent who discusses his or her baby's behaviour in minute detail over dinner will find that the subject quickly changes as eyes glaze over.

'Gradually it dawns on you that it is just "not on". You dissolve instantly into a non-person. Since your day is taken up with babies it is pretty hard to delve into your brain for something interesting to say about a film (the last time you saw one was 'Before Baby' and it has long since receded into the mists of maternal amnesia). It is a relief to meet up with other parents who are happy to compare stories about sleepless nights and nappies. Without even noticing we have started to build up a completely new set of friends – fellow travellers into parenthood.'

Finding someone to talk to who has a baby of roughly the same age can provide you both with company and with space to be with your child. Another mother who is also preoccupied with her child may be happy just to be in the same room with you, making desultory conversation, but without expecting your full attention. Since she is going through the experience at the same time as you she will also take a much greater interest in your baby's progress. This process of comparison (often seen merely as competitiveness) provides you with the most useful source of information you can get about child development as well as genuinely reciprocal support when the going gets rough. Be wary though about how you give advice and how you receive it. This is what one mother felt about 'friendly advice':

'The last child was very unpredictable with solids – a lot of patience was required. I found that the patience only ran out when there were other mothers around busy giving their opinions as to what I should do. I could see he was a healthy boy, full of energy and putting on weight even though he wasn't eating solids.'

If a friend whose baby sleeps angelically most of the day tries to tell you how to make your fractious little screamer behave the same way, you are unlikely to feel grateful for the advice. It will almost certainly *feel* patronising even if it is very well meant. It probably won't help much even if you do listen. She cannot provide you with a solution because she hasn't experienced the problem (even if she thinks she has). What you want to hear is how other mothers with the same problem have coped.

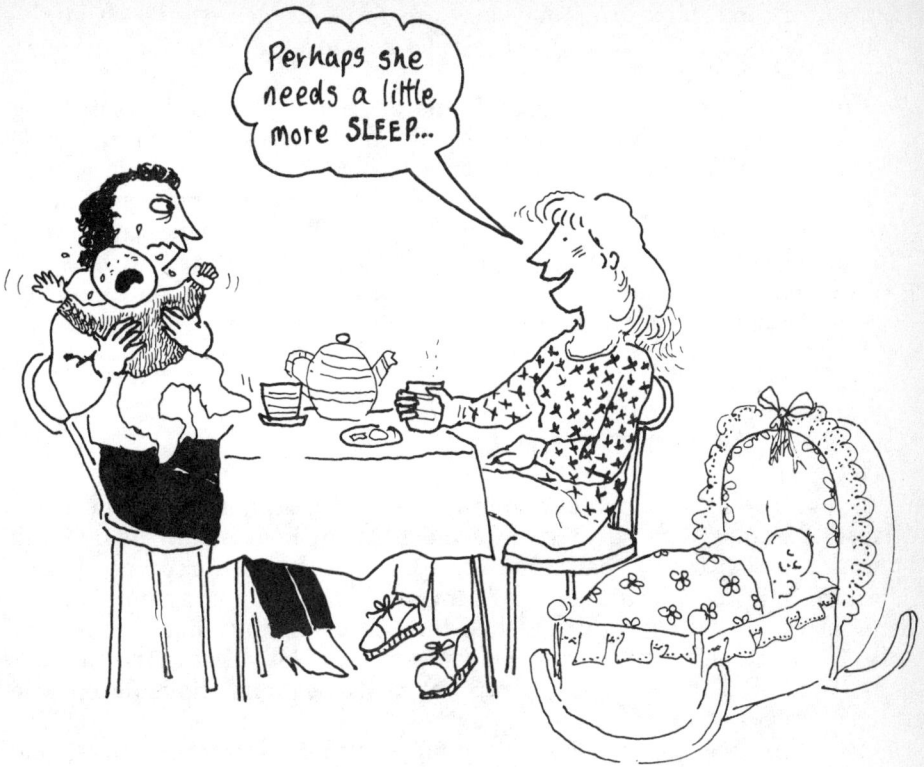

'I think the most comforting advice comes from people who say: "I know what you are going through, my child did that too." Then you feel free to ask what approaches they used to solve the problem. It is information shared by equals. Not advice dished out by someone who feels superior.'

Postnatal support groups, mother and baby clubs or One O'Clock clubs are all places where parents of babies can meet. There may also be toy libraries where you have the added bonus of borrowing toys suitable for your child's particular stage of development. If you don't know what is available locally, ask your health visitor or enquire at your Baby Clinic. Organisations like Cry-sis, (see Help Organizations, p. 210) have special support groups for parents of crying babies, and health visitors in your area may have set up a group for parents experiencing sleeping problems with their children.

Fathers who care for small babies may have greater problems than mothers because many of the existing groups are quite hostile to men. Just as women experience 'sexual harrassment' in an all-male working environment, women are quite capable of dishing out the same treatment to a man who they feel has invaded a female stronghold. Even where women make a real effort to welcome fathers, it may be hard for a father to talk about the problems he is experiencing, in case this is seen as evidence of his inate inability to do a mother's job.

Men do bring different skills and different approaches to the mothering role. They have after all been trained differently. Just as women in a male world derive a great deal of support from meeting together with other women to discuss common problems, men caring for small children may get similar support from meeting other men doing this job. The numbers of men who take on the sole care of a baby or young child for all, or part, of the week are still small but it may well be worth putting a card up in your clinic or in a shop window asking if there are other men with babies who would like to get in touch.

WHEN A PARTNERSHIP ENDS

When parents stop being able to communicate with each other partnerships collapse. I do not propose to go into much detail here about divorce and separation except to say that children suffer, and they also recover. It is as important to acknowledge their suffering as it is to put energy into helping them get over it. If you have reached the point of being unable to talk to each other without fighting you may need help. Not necessarily for your sakes (you will find a way of coping) but for the sake of the children who are part of both of you.

An uninvolved third party could help you to deal with the anger and bitterness you feel and help you sort out a common plan for the care of your children. With an agreed plan for access, or shared care, you can both put your energies into letting your children know, as concretely as you can, that no matter what happens, they will always be loved and cared for and safe. Relate (which used to be the Marriage Guidance Council) provides counselling for couples, married or not, whether you are committed to staying together or determined to part.

Your children will grieve, they will want to go on hoping that you will get back together, they may even try to engineer it. They will hate it if they hear you being unkind about each other and they will feel bewildered and divided if you try to get them to take sides. They do not want to be part of your quarrels. They may be furiously angry at you for upsetting their lives or they may turn their anger inwards, fearing that they are responsible for this catastrophe.

They have a right to their anger and they have reason to be angry with you. Your child may start to have tantrums or nightmares. He may hate you to leave him in the morning or he may become hostile and surly. Try to find ways in which he can say the things that are on his mind. Sometimes his fears may seem so enormous that he is literally afraid to express them.

'She wouldn't talk about what was happening until I said, what is the thing you fear most? She said I am afraid that something will happen to you and I will have to look after Joanne (her baby sister) by myself. When I explained that, even if something did happen to me, her dad would look after her and that, if something happened to him, her uncle and aunt would take over, she started to relax. She needed to know that her future was secure whatever happened.'

A loss that is just covered over doesn't go away. It lies there festering, digging a deep hole in our self-confidence. If your child remains cheerful and apparently unconcerned, don't just breathe a sigh of relief and think you got away lightly. Try to get her to talk about it. Tell other people who care for her what is going on so that they too can help to rebuild the hole in the net of her security.

Sometimes it is hard to remember that our children have relationships with the people who care for them which are quite separate from our own. We owe it to them to try and allow that relationship to continue. Adults who have not been tied to their children by the bonds of biology may find that society does not give them much encouragement to keep in touch. The ex-lover does not have a big claim on a child in the eyes of the law. Yet if a child has a relationship with an adult, his or her presence will be missed. Taking on parental responsibility is not just a matter of helping the other parent – it is a longterm commitment to a child, a trust which should not be betrayed.

Chapter 2

LEARNING THROUGH LIVING

When I was One,
I had just begun.

When I was Two,
I was nearly new.

When I was Three,
I was not quite me.

When I was Four,
I was not much more.

When I was Five,
I was just alive.

But now I am Six, I'm as clever as clever.
I think I'll be six now for ever and ever.
(A. A. Milne, *Now We Are Six*)

Children are programmed to learn. From the moment they are born they are drinking in everything around them and pushing at the limits of their physical capacities. As parents most of us are eager to help that process along, or at the very least to avoid hampering it. If we want to help our children effectively we have to start from where they are. To do that we have to learn from them.

PARENT DEVELOPMENT

Getting to know your baby

The parents of newborn babies (particularly first ones) are often described as 'doting' or obsessive. More blasé and experienced parents observe with amusement as a new mother or father jumps up every time the baby squeaks or sighs. The parents of a one-year-old are not intimately concerned with the developmental progress of a newborn – they have moved on. You, of course, are quite right to be obsessive. Without that minute interest you will not be able to learn about your baby's unique pattern of behaviour. You will not be able to learn how best to react to her needs. You need two things: enough time alone with your child to be able to learn that rhythm intimately and the company of other parents, at the same stage as you, whose experience can provide you with more information that you can get from your child alone.

Only you can judge how much time you need alone with your child. If you are finding it impossible to come to terms with your baby's changing needs you might need more time than you are getting. If you are overrun with friends and relations who want your attention, you may need the courage to be firm and say no. If you are a single parent you have a dilemma. You want company and you want to be alone with your baby. It is hard to cater for both these needs. It may help if you make a clear plan to prioritise your needs on some days and the baby's needs on others. (see 'Getting Support', p. 10)

From the very first hours after birth, parents and babies start the job of working out a partnership. Psychologist Rudolph Schaffer described the process in his book *Mothering* (Fontana, 1977):

> *'An adult generally wants to know roughly what response he will produce with any particular form of stimulation. When he picks up the baby, boisterously swings him through the air and bounces him up and down he does so in the belief that the baby will respond by gurgling with delight. Whether that happens, though, depends entirely on how sensitively he read the baby's initial state, for under some conditions that treatment will produce screams of protest and howls of rage.'*

The job is made harder, as well as more fascinating, because babies are not all the same. They do not emerge as blank canvasses for us to write upon – they have different temperaments. Take cuddliness, for example.

> *'My first child found cuddling an interference which stopped him reaching out to grab at life. I had to wait for those moments just before he dropped off to sleep when he would allow his head to drop on my shoulder or lock his arms around my neck. Perversely I enjoyed his early illnesses when he would let me hold him close. I had looked forward to cuddling and was a bit disappointed but it was clearly not to do with lack of love. He just had other ways of expressing the way he felt about us. My second is quite different, a real cuddler. Seeing how much we both enjoy it, the older one has started, occasionally, to give it a try but after a couple of minutes he is up and off to do something more interesting.'*

Schaffer found that:

Most mothers, however surprised they may be initially by non-cuddling, quickly adjust and find other ways of furthering the relationship. It is only when they are too inflexible, or interpret the baby's behaviour as rejection, that trouble can arise from a mis-match.'

Parents of non-cuddlers are just starting a little earlier than most on the way to understanding that children have needs of their own. We have to learn to respond to the way our children *already are.*

CRYING BABIES

Some babies and parents instantly 'click'. They fall into ways of being which work from day one. The baby sleeps happily, coos when awake, only cries when hungry and then feeds happily. For others, the task of accommodation is hard work. Sometimes it is because we are too anxious about 'doing it right' to take our cue from the baby.

'The screaming of the early weeks was awful. I would leave her crying for a minute and then ring her father to say "I've left her crying. Is that OK?" and then I would rush back. I needed a lot of support from him, and I got it. But there was a limit to what he could do over the phone.'

In the end this mother discovered that her baby was tired and all the rocking and jiggling was stopping her from sleeping. Once she realised just how much sleep this particular baby actually needed (see Sleep, Chapter 4) everything started to fall into place. The baby slept when she was tired and responded happily to her parents when she was awake. The screaming stopped.

All babies cry occasionally, no matter how sensitively we read their behaviour. You may learn very quickly how best to respond to the cries or you may find that nothing you do helps. Don't assume that you are the problem. Some babies just seem to be unsettled for a period every day for the first three months. As one mother said:

'With my first baby I got upset. By 8.30 every evening I would be so exhausted I would just take her to bed with me. The second child followed the same pattern. At about three weeks he started to get unsettled and cry every evening between 5 pm and about 11 pm. I just decided I would have to cope until it stopped. It meant no social life for three months but it didn't seem a lot to pay in a lifetime. Just remind yourself that this period doesn't last.'

Unsettled periods can be coped with fairly easily if your child wakes up bright as a button in the morning and gurgles her way through the first part of the day. However, some babies go on crying inconsolably for hours no matter how sensitively their parents respond to their needs. Some may just be more touchy than others, more easily startled and generally sensitive to loud noises, cold, or handling.

There is also some evidence that these unhappy babies may have been affected by difficult birth experiences. Sheila Kitzinger, in her book *The Crying Baby* (Viking, 1989), suggests that they may have been affected by events occurring before they were born. She found that the mothers of persistently crying babies were more likely to have been through episodes of extreme stress during pregnancy (not just everyday worry – external problems over which they had no control). She suggests that these babies are born with a high level of anxiety which they need to discharge through crying, and she advises:

> *'When you realise that things that happened even before your baby was born – circumstances you could not change, although you very much wanted to – may have affected the baby, and understand that these were the same things that caused you distress in pregnancy, you will no longer feel responsible for, and guilty about, the crying. It is not faulty mothering that is making your baby cry; instead it is the out-pouring of response to a stress you both shared.'*

Having understood that they are not the *cause* of their babies' distress, Kitzinger hopes that these parents will find it easier to accept the crying as part of how their baby is – something to be 'read' along with everything else and not merely something to be stopped at all costs. That acceptance may not make the early months much easier to live through, but it may help parents to focus on the positive moments, not only on the crying.

A very wakeful or crying baby is exhausting. It is often hard to find enough time in the day to think about how you are coping, let alone consider how your baby is developing. You just want some peace. The best help anyone can give you is not by advising how you can cope, but by giving you a break in which *you* can think about how to cope.

Having a baby who is hard to comfort does have its compensations. All that rocking and stroking, pram rides and music, are providing masses of stimulation. This sort of baby is forcing you to concentrate on his needs and if you can find the peace of mind to give back half of what is demanded of you, when the crying stops, you will have a baby whom you know intimately. A father, interviewed in *The Crying Baby*, described the process like this:

> *'At first I tried to grasp everything with logic. I would go through a mental checklist to see if the baby had everything and failed to understand why she went on crying. Then I began to try different kinds of behaviour, approaching her with feelings, and then I began to understand her. Suddenly there are no more rules. What calms today may not work tomorrow.'*

(Crying is also discussed in Chapter 4. Cry-sis! is a self-help organisation for the parents of crying babies. It is listed in the Help section at the back of the book.)

WHAT DO THEY NEED?

Learning to 'read' our children never stops being important. As children get older they can be reasoned with and asked to explain what they need and want, but the art of 'mind reading' will still be a great help – knowing when your child is too hungry, tired or simply distracted to concentrate; sensing when an activity is about to disintegrate into a squabble; divining whether your child doesn't want to get in the water because a) she is afraid, b) the water is cold, c) she wants you to stay with her until she is in.

If we can be sufficiently 'tuned in' to get it right more often than not, our children will find learning and growing a pleasure, and so will we. If we are totally unable to tune in, *we* will find the process agonising. Our children will probably take what they want and leave the rest (unless we resort to force). Most of us get it wrong some of the time. Often it is because we are

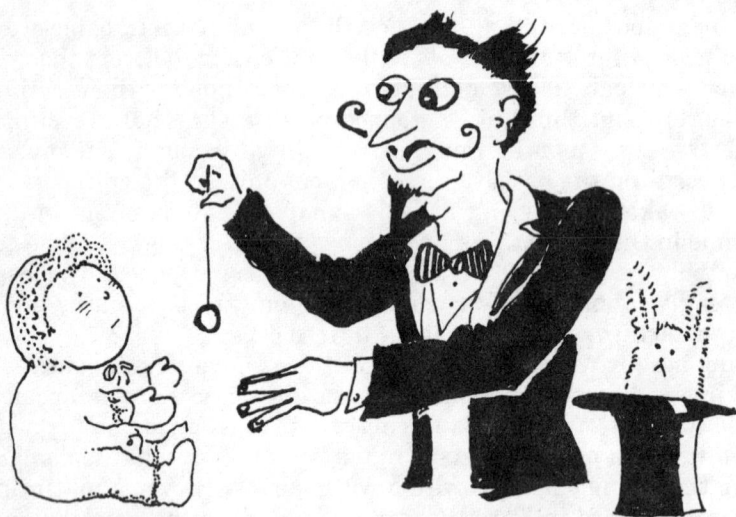

The Great Parento
~ Juggler ~ Magician ~ Mind-Reader

looking at learning from our point of view, not theirs. Once it stops being fun, they will probably switch off. The time when we are most likely to make learning a chore is when *we* feel unhappy or anxious about it. A primary school teacher who spent most of the first five years of her children's lives at home with them had this to say:

> *'If you feel bad about an area it is probably best to leave it alone and just do the stuff you get a kick out of doing yourself.'*

That seems to me to be pretty good advice, but it is not enough to think only about what we want to teach our children or what they are capable of learning. We have to think also about what is useful for our children to know. Some parents feel the need to fill their children's heads with facts as an insurance policy against future educational failure.

At the extreme end this kind of parental ambition results in the 'hot-housing' of babies and children which is becoming common in America. According to Glen Doman, the guru of the hot-housers:

> *'Parents can give their babies the degree of genius that each individual baby will have by the amount and variety of auditory, and tactile stimulation they give the child and the judicious use of the frequency, intensity and duration with which they give it.'*

He teaches parents to programme their children from birth, using 'flash cards' containing facts and figures which they manage to store and to regurgitate on demand. The feats of skill are astonishing, for example two-year-olds solving complex mathematical equations, and learning to read before they can talk. Psychiatrist Martin James is extremely critical of this approach and feels sure it can only produce 'more mad children':

> *'What a baby can learn usefully is different from what it can be taught. You can teach it anything, but there are other things which we should do at eighteen months that are more important. A baby should be learning about touching, stroking and feeling.'*

In the early years, he would argue, our children should be learning primarily about loving and being loved. We might think that our children's formal education and economic security is the most important thing for their future, but will they agree? After all, as James wisely observes: 'It's hell to have a relationship with someone who can read about making love without being able to make love.'

During your baby's first year she will be growing and changing almost daily (see 'What children can do', pp. 25–34). Within weeks it will no longer be enough to feed, change and rock her. She will want entertainment: new things to look at and hear, other babies and children to watch, exciting things to handle and touch. But most of all she will want you – her parents, brothers and sisters and carers. She will want your touch, your voice, your smell, the ever-changing expressions on your faces. If you hold and touch your baby as much as she wants to be held and touched, it will never be too much. When she is happy and alert you can never talk too much, sing too much or show her too many ducks or flowers in the park, blossom on the trees, or branches swaying in the breeze.

Bathing, changing and feeding are not just events that break up the day, they are the times when you can be most intimate with your child.

'It was important to me that my child should be strong. I believe that physical things support mental and physical development. To start with I did lots of stretching her hands and arms and massage using coconut oil. Oiling her skin was part of the ritual of bathing because black skin gets very dry in this climate. We also spent a lot of time together skin on skin, just being physically close. I gave Ebony what I would have wanted for myself. To be lovingly held and cuddled. In giving you get some back.'

In the first year the only thing your baby needs to learn from you is that she is safe and loved. The rest of the learning she will do for herself – as long as you let her. That learning will be about everything: the child who crawls over and switches on the television set at ten months old has not been told how to do it – she has worked it out just by watching.

'I was holding my son on my hip and he desperately wanted to press the buttons on the washing machine. It was switched off on the wall so when he pressed the button nothing happened. He immediately pointed at the wall switch. He knew how to switch on the machine and knew that I hadn't completed the sequence.'

A two-year-old who expertly rocks a 'baby' in his arms and then carefully tucks him into bed has not read the instructions – he learned it by copying you. If you kiss and hold him he learns that kissing and holding feels good and he will crawl on to Grandad's lap in the hope of more. By two years old he will be greeting other well loved friends with a kiss and a hug too. If he didn't learn about kissing and hugging his life would be the poorer for it.

We teach our children to notice the sunset or to tell a dandelion from a daffodil, we may teach our children about the names and 'strip' of every club in the football league. The things we care about we pass on, by showing, by talking or just by doing everyday things. Most parents also want to teach some of the basic steps towards formal learning.

'How can you not teach things? You are answering their questions, showing and naming and explaining things all the time. A lot of their learning is through repetition but it is voluntary – asking you to repeat until it sinks in. I don't think you can force it, but if you are open to it, and have time and patience for it, it must help. Some concepts

– colours, numbers – you can prepare the ground for, but they will
get there when they are ready. When they see it, recognise it.'

Certainly our children will get a better start in their educational lives if, by
the time they start school at five, they have already been introduced to
books and can tell the difference between text and pictures, and if they are
beginning to understand what numbers *mean* and have had some experience
of tasks such as colouring-in and cutting which give them some control over
a pencil or other simple tools. None of these lessons need to be pressured.
They can be picked up in the course of everyday life, while discovering the
feeling of the sun on their backs, wind in their hair, the joys of flying through
the air on a swing, whizzing down a slide, digging in the sand. It doesn't
require particular skills, or full-time mothering.

'Just around two she started to see letters in the world, Z's in the
wrought iron railings. She made it clear to me that she was already
interested in words and symbols. If you listen and watch, your children
will tell you what they are interested in.'

Failing is bad for the brain

For a young child learning is a game. A three-year-old who asks to cut up
an old magazine with a pair of scissors doesn't know that this is an important
learning activity. She is enjoying it just as much as the game she played
earlier giving tea to her dolls. Learning stops being a game when it becomes
competitive, or when parents introduce pressure. If it stops being fun, your
child may simply lose interest.

Two- and three-year olds want to win all the time. There is no pleasure
in failure so if they sense that they are failing in some way they will usually
cheat, scream, or change the subject. Children love being asked questions.
They find it exciting and challenging – but only if they get the answers
right. If they cannot win they won't want to play.

'My first child clearly had a mathematical bent. He learned and
understood about numbers when he was three and would enjoy little
problems like working out how many children were going to be coming
for tea and, if one went home, how many would be left. I tried the
same games with his younger brother but he took far longer to
understand the concepts involved. He just pretended he hadn't heard
the question.'

By being tested before he was ready this child was already learning, at the
tender age of three, that numbers are a trap to be wary of. If we want to
help our children to learn without stress, and to enjoy learning, we have to
make sure that they always win.

'We used to ask a group of children to "name" colours. Tahiba and James knew all their colours already and would compete to be the first to shout out the answer. Matthew and Ruth were not yet sure enough to get it right. After a couple of goes they started making wild guesses or refused to join in at all. Testing them in this way was making them anxious about the whole issue.'

If we set up learning games in which there are winners, we also create losers. No child will be helped by early education if this has simply been a lesson in failure. A better approach would be to use more oblique ways of testing the children's knowledge. Casually asking what colour crayon or paper a child would like or asking her to pass a particular colour gives us the same information about the child's progress without exposing her knowledge, or lack of it, so clearly. Another way of testing without asking questions is to pretend to make mistakes yourself, for example, trying to put a piece of a jigsaw puzzle in upside down and then letting the child correct you.

Letting the other one win

While we don't want to teach our children to fail, we do need to introduce the concept of sharing and turn-taking and learning to understand another person's point of view. To some extent these are all lessons in *not* winning, but we can look at them more positively as lessons in the value of winning together, which is what cooperation is all about.

The issue usually arises first over 'sharing'. At around two years old children very often become fiercely possessive and will fight viciously for a toy. Teaching sharing is hard but worthwhile. It is a perfect opportunity to help a child understand the value of cooperation: 'I'll let you play with my toy if I can play with something of yours.' Children nearly always find it harder to part with possessions in their own home. What they own is part of their sense of territory. In a playgroup or nursery they quickly begin to learn that toys are 'in common'. If a dispute develops the toy will simply be removed and nobody will get it.

At home it may help if each child has some possessions which are indisputably his or her own as well as ones which are for sharing. If a child comes to visit the special toys can then be put away and some sense of territory preserved. Your child may then get a sense of pride and pleasure out of allowing a friend to share these special toys as long as he is clear that he has complete control over the decision to share and that the toy can be removed again if he becomes anxious about it. Children do not grow out of possessiveness (after all, how happy are *you* about sharing your records, or your clothes?) but as they get more interested in playing with other children they work out a balance between the need to keep safe and the need to share.

Another way of teaching the value of turn-taking is through card and board games. If a three-year-old plays Snap, for example, she will learn that the game can only work if she occasionally allows the other person to win. To begin with that might just mean that she shares out the cards she has just won. Working out when to expect more 'give and take' is, once again, a question of knowing your own child, or being sensitive to the children in your care.

PLEASURABLE PARENTING

Of all the parents who talked or wrote of their experiences of parenting only one lamented that:

> 'It was a pleasure, but time was a problem. I always felt I should have done more.'

This was a fulltime mother who felt, presumably, that she had to take full responsibility for everything her child learned. There is no law which says that children should learn only from their parents. Indeed I have found that any of my attempts at teaching very quickly became tense. I have always been happy to leave much of my children's learning to other carers. The privilege of a working mother who shares her child care with others is that she can pick and choose. We can do the bits we like and leave the rest to others.

> 'Frankly I do not get a kick out of standing in a freezing cold wintry park watching my children gambol happily on the slides. If it had been all up to me I would have had to choose between discomfort and guilt because I believe that children should be able to gambol in wintry parks. Thank goodness (and Linda) that I have been able to leave the winter gambolling to others while still getting the pleasure of snuggling up in a warm room reading stories.'

We can't all pick and choose and not all of us want or need to. A parent who can treat each new day as an adventure shared (letting the washing-up pile up in the sink and ignoring the unhoovered stairs) will be getting every ounce of pleasure out of parenting. Peggy Wynn, grandmother of six, looks back to her early mothering days during the war:

> 'How many dozens of times one of those older working-class women (in the Women's Cooperative Guild) would say to me "Now make the most of it love, it never comes again, and once they are gone they are gone." They took all the backwards looking and forward looking out

of me for the time being and taught me to make a party of every day.
Even a trip for the rations could be memorable if I remembered to
linger over the garden which had a dozen gnomes in it.'

These first five years are indeed precious. Though my older child had been
cared for away from me (for part of the day) since babyhood I, like so many
other mothers, had a lump in my throat the day he started big school. I was
crying for the end of an era. It was the first day of *real* separation when I
knew that his life was starting to take on a shape of its own and I would
have to start the long painful job of learning how to let go – but that's
another story.

A child's right to grow

Over the last few years I have watched more than a dozen small children
growing and playing together on a regular basis. Some came from African or Carribbean backgrounds, others were white, most were middle
class, some were not. The most accomplished talker could hold a conversation before her second birthday. Physically she was probably the slowest child, with a real fear of climbing. The only child who could recognise
written numbers and some words before he turned three was also the
slowest talker.

Our children did not develop at the same speed. Some made leaps
forward, others moved forward more slowly. There were some gender
differences (see 'Will boys be boys?', pp. 34–7) but an additional factor
which certainly affected their development was stress. Several children
had to cope with a high degree of stress in their first three years: parents
separating or dealing with problems at work, or new babies being born.
Some reacted by withdrawing, perhaps taking comfort from quiet, concentrated activity. Others kicked out or regressed in some way. The
support that the parents were able to give each other and the security
provided by the group and workers meant that these stresses, in most
cases, were short lived. The children came through and their developmental progress continued or caught up.

Most children do not have the security of a group they belong to
which can dilute the stress of their domestic circumstances, when the
going gets rough. They just have to cope, at second hand, with everything
their parents go through. Children who are coping with daily stress from
birth will not have had the opportunity to stretch out and find out the
best that they can do. They will be starting off their educational lives
with a real disadvantage.

A society which believed in the right of all children to the best
possible start in life would do everything in its power to relieve stress
on small children. Instead it allows large numbers of parents to live in

poverty, sits back whilst many mothers suffer chronic depression, and does virtually nothing to alleviate the everyday strain of racism.

Small children want to learn, they want to grow up, they want to communicate but they need adult help. With the best will in the world parents cannot give that help if the burden of their life saps all their energy and the effort of existence takes all their time. Alleviating family poverty, and providing nurseries and play centres so that all children have access to safe and stress-free places to grow, should be top of the list of priorities for any civilised society.

WHAT CHILDREN CAN DO

The first year

During her first year, your baby will be spending most of her time working out how to make her body do what she wants it to do. Some new-born babies find the constant stimulation too much to cope with and are alarmed even by their own limbs moving in the air without the reassuring pressure of fluid and their mother's body. A jumpy, crying baby might like to be wrapped tight in a shawl, particularly at sleeping times, to reduce the amount of new stimulation to a level he can cope with. He can hear even before he is born and will respond particularly to anything with a body rhythm.

Babies like music and sound with a human pattern: the recorded sound of a heartbeat will often soothe a crying baby. African drum rhythms seem to have a similar effect. Lullabies and work songs have been used down the centuries to soothe and they work just as well today.

Your baby's first achievement will be to make her face move into a smile. The response will of course be overwhelming and she will probably want to go on smiling just to see you copy her. She has always been able to see your face while you feed her and gradually her field of focus broadens to take in far more of the world. She still likes face-shaped things best and will smile at almost anything that is round with two eyes. She also likes detailed patterns:

'I found out quite by accident that the wallpaper in the bathroom had a magical effect on Ruth. It was white with a small dotty pattern. If she was crying I needed only to take her in there and she would stare mesmerised at the wall – seemed a little odd at the time.'

Within weeks that little head which flopped onto your shoulder will start

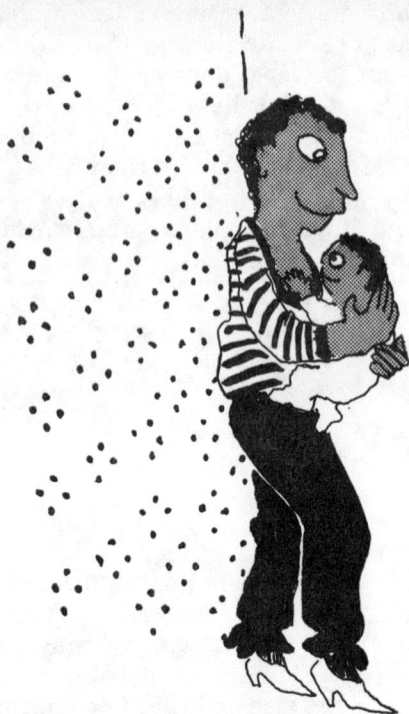

to come under control so that the beady eyes can peer over the top and take in the world. You will start to hear babbling noises now which are the beginnings of speech. It is never too soon to talk back. She enjoys listening to the sounds of a human voice better than anything. We talk to our babies almost instinctively in ways they are most likely to respond to. Put even the least child-oriented person with a young baby and they will move close, speak higher than usual, and simplify their speech, using sound patterns that the baby enjoys and tries to copy. Baby-talk is not evidence of the brain-softening effect of parenthood – it is an important first step to teaching your child to talk. If you force yourself to talk only as you would to an adult you will be going against your own gut feeling of how to talk to your baby – trust your gut. As your child learns to talk, and to understand, you will automatically start using more complex sentences and lowering the tone of your voice.

By four months your baby's neck muscles will be sturdy enough to support her head so that she can peep over the top of her crib or carrycot. Now she can make some use of her hands to wave a rattle or spoon and thoroughly mess up your first attempts to spoonfeed her! She can sit for a short time, with her back well supported, in a high chair or moulded baby seat, so now she has a better view of what is going on. She may well have started to cut her first tooth.

By six months many things have been achieved: she can reach out and grab the hot cup of tea you left too near and she can get her own beaker to her mouth and drink unaided. She may well be able to roll off the bed if you turn your back. Sitting, well propped up with cushions, she can find things in a 'treasure basket' full of interesting (and safe) objects to chew and examine. (Elinor Goldschmied discussed this in 'Play and learning in the first year of life', *Babies in Day Care*, The Daycare Trust, 1989)

You can make your own treasure basket. Start collecting as soon as your baby is born. The objects should be safe. Nothing small enough to swallow or choke on; nothing with sharp edges and nothing that cannot be relatively easily cleaned or thrown out. Look for different textures, colours and shapes: wooden spoon, lemon squeezer, a few small pieces of carpet samples in different colours, a marble egg, a small square of sand paper, a wooden block and a bell. Keep changing the objects to keep things interesting.

She cannot say any words yet but she can already have a 'conversation'. If you copy the sounds she makes, she will stop, listen to you, and then repeat them. She will enjoy rhymes, particularly if they have a good explosive end, or actions to go with them.

Ten little sausages frying in a pan,
one went POP, the other went BANG. (clap hands)
Eight little sausages frying in a pan,
one went POP, the other went BANG, etc.

Peek-a-boo is a game played all over the world and always loved. For a baby it is enough just to cover your face with your hands and then remove them and smile. Variations on this theme will probably produce peals of joyful laughter for years.

By nine months she can sit up unsupported, which makes it much easier to play, but she will still be dropping everything and then yelling at you to give it back if it rolls away. If you put her regularly on the floor to play she will start making efforts to retrieve things herself. She will still enjoy a treasure basket full of interesting playthings and she will get great pleasure out of playing in water or with sand (try to stop her eating it!) Old detergent bottles and plastic cups can turn bathtime into the greatest pleasure of the day. Water play will go on being a favourite for years.

She may well have developed a special relationship with a teddy, doll, or piece of cloth which she likes to keep with her at all times. Her 'fine motor' skills are developing. That means she can pick out the peas in her dinner if you don't mash them in.

She will be learning to crawl which means she will be permanently filthy and able to find (and eat) all sorts of tiny objects that you hadn't noticed under the table. Older brothers or sisters will find her spoiling their toys and be unable to resist taking revenge. Fortunately she is now tough enough to withstand a certain amount of sibling bullying. She will also learn how to pull herself up to standing – a feat she will almost certainly want to demonstrate every time she wakes up at night. By the end of her first year she may even have taken her first wobbly steps alone, but each child is different. Your child may be getting around very well on her bottom or knees and show little interest in walking for another six months.

Listen for those first words. 'Dada' will almost certainly be the first sound (which is probably why dads are called Dad – it makes them feel important to be the first person named). Then watch out for 'mama' or 'ema'. Another early sound is 'ca' which pretty soon gets attached to car or cat, and the game of labelling has begun. Some labels will sound nothing like the word you know, and you may find yourself learning your baby's language as he learns yours. This is a good time to introduce books with simple colourful pictures of household objects for her to practise naming.

When I was One I had just begun

In the second year effort goes into improving on the skills learned in the first year.

Walking will move on from wobbling to toddling. By the middle of the year, a reasonably seasoned walker will be coping with stairs, and by the end of the year running will not look such a precarious activity and your baby may even kick a ball at the same time. She will enjoy pushing a cart or baby buggy and 'riding' a pushalong bike. This newfound skill with arms and legs may turn your child into a climber. All children climb – some climb a lot more than others so beware of wobbly bookcases.

Hands become far more useful. At the start of the year they can be used for conveying a spoon to the mouth, for squidging play dough and putting objects in and out of boxes and bowls. Towards the end of the year eye-hand coordination will have improved so that your baby can post shapes through holes if she wants to. Posting real letters is even more fun. Given a pencil and paper she will probably be able to make a few marks and feel pretty good about it. Watch out – her skilful hands can now open doors. Throwing has become a good game, but not always with balls and not always in the right place.

Words spoken early on may disappear and then return later as talking begins to develop. To begin with single words will be heard, often connected with food, and the word 'no' is almost certain to be used – accurately. As the year progresses the number of words will increase, though a stranger will find them very difficult to understand.

'As far as speech was concerned it was different for each child. Our first boy was very talkative when he was nine months old – he could repeat certain syllables but then everything vanished and he only started talking again just before his second birthday. Looking back I suppose I was anxious. Most of his little friends could communicate fairly well by then. Our second boy started speaking when he was just over a year and could speak correct sentences. With the other two I stopped worrying. One started speaking at eighteen months and the other looks like he will take after his first brother.'

When I was Two I was nearly new

At the end of the second year legs and arms are taken for granted. They work – effortlessly. Your baby is a whirlwind of activity, moving from one experience to another. She will need space. If you haven't got it at home, she will be constantly clamouring to go to the park so that she can run and jump freely or ride her push-along bike, but try to get her to walk to nursery in the morning and you may have a battle on your hands! She wants to walk when and where *she* wants to.

Hands need more working on if they are to do what the brain wants them to. A two-year-old will find it hard to coordinate her hand movements well enough to cut a piece of paper, though she will almost certainly want to try, and by the end of the year she will probably be managing quite well. Playing with dough or sand will help her to learn the effective use of her hands.

Play dough is cheap to make and can be kept in an airtight container for months. Take two cups of flour, one of salt, one of water (with colouring in it) and two tablespoons of oil. Knead it together and then warm it gently in a pan until it forms a soft, mouldable lump.

Building will have become an absorbing activity. Towers of bricks (or food tins) can be built and knocked down. Puzzles can provide a wonderful way of playing with your child as well as encouraging eye-hand coordination. But let her lead the way.

'Rose wouldn't do puzzles and she was not the least bit interested in putting different shapes through different holes. The round one was all right – it was easy, but she could not see any reason for putting any effort into something which clearly had no meaning for her. Then one day, she was about two and a half I think, she took a puzzle off the table, went to the other side of the room with her back to everyone else, sat down and put the puzzle together unaided.'

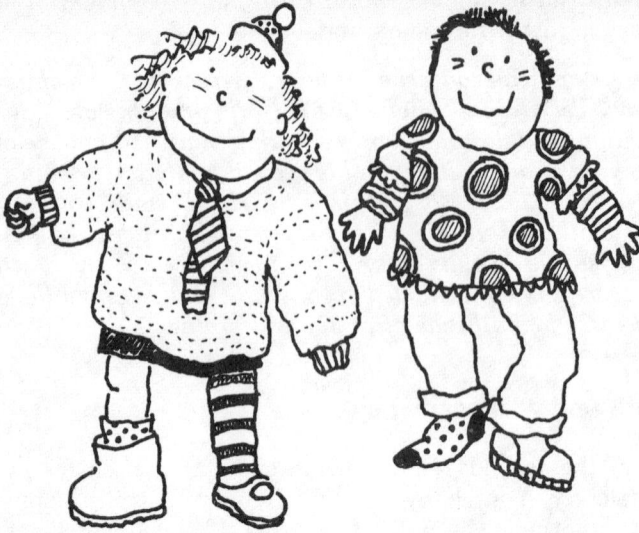

Dressing will become a useful activity as well as a game. By the middle of the year she will have the skill to do most of it herself, if not the inclination. (I know one boy who is a dab hand at lego but simply refuses to dress himself. It clearly doesn't interest him yet.) Don't expect a two-year-old to be able to cope with buttons or zips. She may insist on choosing what clothes she wears, and you will have to brace yourself to accept some eccentricity if you want her to develop this independence. She may also start to get choosy about food, insisting on having it presented exactly as she likes it and turning up her nose at things she is not familiar with.

At the start of this year the gap between what your child knows, and what she can make you understand, will seem frustratingly wide. Her understanding of language is far greater than her ability to use it. She will say something, which to her is perfectly clear, and you won't understand. (Brothers and sisters can be good interpreters.) She probably thinks you should try harder. Towards the end of the year she will be holding conversations not just with you but with herself, because this is the year for make-believe. She may spend long periods of time totally absorbed with a game of mummies and daddies, cars or dressing up or some other fantasy modelled on the life of adults. If she spends time with other children regularly they will be included in the game but she can quite happily play all the parts herself.

My two-year-old daughter told everyone she had a mouse living under her bed. She gave this mouse a life of its own, and took it everywhere with her.'

Fantasy games vary and so do the children who play them. Some require nothing but imagination, speech and a couple of pieces of cloth. Others weave their fantasies around toys. Pushing toy cars up and down a ramp is as much a fantasy of being a grown-up as playing with dolls. Some can sustain fantasy play for long periods while others cannot play alone for ten minutes. You cannot change the way a child plays but you can influence it. A reluctant builder may happily use lego to build her baby a bed and a child who shows little interest in dolls may be encouraged to copy nurturing behaviour if you give him a clearer goal – perhaps nursing a sick teddy.

Most two-year-olds are ready to listen to simple stories though they will probably need pictures to look at to keep their interest. Attention span varies enormously.

> *'This child will listen to three books in a row and then demand more. Her brother would get impatient halfway through the first book and attempt to turn over pages in order to see the picture on the next page before I had finished reading the last one.'*

When I was Three I was not quite me

Your three-year-old will be looking for ways of increasing her knowledge. She can talk and walk, she has always wanted to 'know' everything, but now that enquiring gets more urgent. Some children do most of their learning through observation.

> *'Alan didn't ask many questions. He would go quiet and store things away. Then, perhaps a couple of days later, he would ask something out of the blue that seemed completely unrelated to anything. It was as though he had sorted a problem out and just wanted the last piece of the jigsaw to make it all fit. He would get furious if I didn't understand exactly what he wanted.'*

With other children the question 'why?' may become a constant refrain and every new piece of information will be squirrelled away.

'Why do I have skin?'

'What colour will I be when I grow up?'

'Will I always be a girl?'

Your child is now doing a lot of labelling and repeating. She discovers that Granny is Mummy's mummy and that introduces the strange idea of Mummy as a baby. She begins to get a sense of where she fits into the structure of things. She may know her street and the name of her town and be starting to work out what that means. She has also discovered the difference between boys and girls and will begin to divide everyone she knows.

> *'John's a boy so he's got a willy. Sue's a girl so she's got a "gina".'*

She is prepared to follow instructions now (though only when it suits her), and can sit at a table and concentrate for long enough to do a fairly complicated puzzle. She will discover the joys of colouring inside the lines rather than scribbling and be able to control a pencil well enough to start drawing. Her first face – a circle with two dots in it – will be a joy for all and hang pinned to the kitchen wall until it curls at the edges. As the year progresses she may add arms and legs.

All that water play will be paying off. Your child will be able to pour her own milk or juice, and know when to stop pouring. Some children will have the dexterity to do up their own buttons and write little wavy lines of 'pretend writing,' and they may be able to trace the outlines of a picture or letter. This manual dexterity varies a great deal from one child to another. If we follow the individual child we can avoid inappropriate pushing before the child is ready. A child who learns to do jigsaws at three is no worse off than the one who did it at two, as long as she has learned the skill happily and at the right time for her.

If your child is not already at a nursery or playgroup now is the time to make sure she gets regular contact with other children. She will be able to make friends now without your intervention and will enjoy having someone to play with. Imaginative games still occupy much of her time and now they are getting even more complex.

She will look at books by herself and probably pretend to read them too by following the pictures. This is an important step on the way to reading, the beginning of understanding about the sequence of a story. You can help her to see that the words and the pictures are separate and that you are reading the words, not just looking at the pictures. She may have learned to count but are you sure she knows what counting is? Some children learn counting as a rhyme and do not understand for quite a while what numbering is for.

> 'As an early talker, Joanne could count at two but it was just a rhyme to her, one day, well after her third birthday, we were sitting at the kitchen table and I put out three cups for her to 'count'. She suddenly clicked that each number had to relate to a separate cup. There was a reason for counting.'

This breakthrough may come very quickly with some children and far more slowly with others. Since *understanding* and feeling safe with numbers is the foundation of all future maths knowledge a little help here might be useful – but don't push it. Counting as you go up and down stairs gives children a real feeling of numbering, counting out biscuits as you share them, counting the places at the table, counting dolls or cars. There are loads of opportunities to repeat the lesson in different ways. Games which involve sorting and grouping help too. Stick with numbers under five until you are absolutely sure she has understood the principles involved. It doesn't matter if you are still trying next year. Better a little understood than a lot jumbled up.

She may also recognise some number symbols and letters, perhaps the letter at the start of her own name. Some parents encourage their children to learn letters and words by labelling everything at home: door, bed, chair, etc. Learning isolated words in this way may not be the way your child's school teaches reading, but as long as you have not introduced any pressure into what has been learned so far, it won't, as teachers used to believe, confuse the child or hold her back. It may not push her forward either.

'My son knew a few words before he started school but he promptly forgot them. His school taught reading in a very integrated way: using story books, not word cards, and these isolated words were simply of no use to him.'

This is a good time to introduce games with rules. Your child will still hate losing but will begin to understand that the person who loses this time may win next. She will also be able to understand about taking turns and following the sequence of the game. There are plenty of games designed specially for small children. Most help develop number skills as well as encouraging symbol recognition, matching and sorting.

When I was Four I was not much more

In the last year before starting school most of the remnants of babyhood disappear. Your child may suddenly change shape, losing the roundness of the earlier years. She will also be beginning to take more control over her life. A childminder said:

'Today Matthew went to the toilet without saying anything then came back and got on with what he was doing. I thought to myself, "That's it!" He's four now, he's gone beyond me. He doesn't need me in the same way.'

This new-found maturity is only partial. Your child will still feel anxious in a new situation, and still needs to know who will pick him up from nursery and who is going to put him to bed, but he is beginning to be able to see things from your point of view too. If you explain that you cannot pick him up today because of a meeting he may moan but he will understand and be able to anticipate if you promise him a treat on Saturday to make up for it.

Your child's skills will be developing rapidly. Cutting and sticking are no longer random activities, they are making pictures. With greater control of a pencil, human shapes are appearing and cars, houses and flowers. Your child may be able to produce letter shapes, although many will be back to front. Lego and other construction games provide scope for quite complex three-dimensional building too. Towards the end of this year you may want to teach your child to ride a bike and swim.

You will need to start preparing your child for the less protected environment of a school where she may be competing with thirty children (or more) for adult attention. Skills such as putting on her own shoes (only the most dextrous four-year-old will manage tieing laces), doing up buttons and eating with a knife and fork will all be useful. However the experience she will find most difficult to adjust to will be the social one of making friends without adult help. A nursery class or playgroup will give your child this experience but a day nursery, with very small numbers of children, will not. Moving from a group of six to a group of thirty will be a shock.

It will be well worthwhile doing a bit of research and making sure that your child meets one or two children who are going to be in her class at school. It may also be worth transferring your child out of a day nursery and into the school nursery for a short period even though it will certainly make life more complicated for you if you are working. If there is no school nursery, or no place available, or you simply cannot cope with the disruption, be prepared to give your child a lot of support in the first school term.

A child who has already been in the school nursery will probably experience little difficulty in making the transition but it is still worthwhile for one or both parents to plan to take a little time off at this stage, if they possibly can, and be available after school to provide love and support if necessary.

WILL BOYS BE BOYS?

If we only give our girls dolls to play with and our boys guns and construction sets we are making sure that they learn different skills which will take them on different routes as they grow up. The girls will go, as they always have, into jobs which are tied to caring for others and are usually low paid and undervalued. The boys will take the other jobs and better pay. The girls may well live more balanced lives, partly in paid work, partly involved in the web of the community, school, friends, home. Boys may grow up to identify mainly as bread-winners still looking to others to provide the comfort and care they have never learned to give.

It is a pattern which should be complementary but too often it isn't. It sets up economic insecurity for women and emotional deprivation for men. If we are to change this cycle children must be given every opportunity to acquire a range of skills, not just those that have been considered suitable for their sex. However it is not just a simple question of giving children 'the right toys'. There are other influences at work.

Among the children I know, the girls generally worked out faster how to use scissors and control a pencil. Boys, on the whole, grasped the point of puzzles earlier and were more likely to build in three dimensions. Girls would use the same bricks but often used them to make borders around things rather than to build structures. These sorts of differences have been quite widely recognised. Any alert teacher, for example, will notice that, in general, girls learn to write faster than boys.

Communication skills are another area of gender difference which has been well researched. Though the boys and girls I have known tended to start talking at roughly the same time, the girls' speech developed faster, and in a far more complex way. They were learning to use speech for more than simply giving and taking instructions.

The boys are generally more active. They climb things, run and jump and shout, just for the sake of doing it. When the girls first started to use their bodies they also enjoyed all these physical things. As they got older they seemed to lose their initial two-year-old boldness about climbing and running whereas the boys' confidence grew. It was almost as though their horizons were already starting to close down as they focussed on elaborate fantasy games.

These gender differences in skill acquisition do exist but they are weaker influences than those of birth order and class. Take language development, for example. Some researchers have noticed that the order a child comes in the family is more important than gender. A first-born boy is likely to develop speech faster than a third-born girl. It is hard to see how such indistinct differences (most of which at an early age favour girls) could lead to the clear gender divisions which are obvious in the way in which even quite small children play.

Rôle division is not a result of skill differences (being good at writing is not a skill widely regarded as necessary for mothering!). As we have already seen, children have an enormous appetite for learning and they learn not only what we tell them but, above all, what they see. Parental influence is very strong. By three a little girl knows that she is a girl 'like Mummy'. She knows what her future will be because she can see Mummy acting it out for her and much of her play is about copying it. Even a mother who goes out to work spends much of the time when she is with her children carrying out specific household tasks.

Boys have no such certainties. Most of them don't *know* what Daddy does because they hardly ever see him doing it. They pretty soon get tired of playing house, because, when all the roles have been allocated, they always get lumbered with playing Dad – and Dad doesn't DO anything. (I know of one little boy who used to fight for the 'baby' rôle. Clearly the rôle of baby is more clearly defined than that of father.) It is not surprising then that these little boys seem to literally run around in circles looking for rôle models and fill the gap with heroes: Superman, Bat Man, Mr T and all the rest.

In spite of the fact that fathers in our society do not provide a visible role model for much of the time, researchers have found that they have more influence than mothers in creating sex roles. Mothers are less concerned about reinforcing the boyishness of their boys and are quite often delighted with assertiveness in their girls. It is often fathers who insist on a little boy's baby curls being cut off because 'everyone thinks he's a girl'.

Girls, who model themselves on the women in their lives, are much freer to move out of the female role. They can play football, wear jeans, and even fight if they wish. It is fathers who want their boys to be 'real men' and their girls to be 'little dolls'. So it is interesting that the children I know who are least sex-defined have fathers who quite consciously do *not* reinforce sex rôles.

The only girl I have encountered who never played with dolls, was cared for mainly by her father (who was totally uninterested in dolls) while her mother was at work. The only boy I have observed playing regularly and intimately with dolls was the quietest amongst a group of bossy girls who to a large extent laid the ground rules for imaginative play. His father is a gentle person who clearly does not react negatively to his son's gentleness. Otherwise most girls liked to play with dolls (just as their mothers had the major care of them) and most of the boys preferred playing with cars (one of the few tasks they ever saw their fathers engage in).

I have watched many mothers forcing themselves, against their own conditioning and education, to deprive their daughters of dolls in the hope that they would take to building instead. But it is hard for us to teach our children to be people that we are not. They are too clever to let us get away with it. Most of these girls nursed teddies instead and were far more interested in drawing and writing than in building. The girls who learned to build were girls who had a parent who was interested in building with them (in every case a father).

The boys, many of whom had initial difficulties with learning to write (just as their sisters had difficulty learning to build), always had massive support in this endeavour from someone who was interested in writing – their mothers. So, in the end, all the boys learn to write. A lot less effort is put into encouraging them to do the other things girls do: to put dolls to bed, to dress up, and to learn how to use speech instead of physical aggression.

Boys model themselves on what the men in their lives actually are, not what they pretend to be. Boys who are brought up without close male models are more likely to learn to be caring than those living closely with men who do not themselves do caring work. Research bears this out. Boys from fatherless homes are often described as being less aggressive and less achievement-oriented.

This 'deviation' from the male model is always described negatively. Caring skills have not been the subject of research and scrutiny. They have not been considered important. No one, it would seem, is interested in what turns men into carers. However much society may have kicked against women doing 'men's jobs' it kicks far harder at the thought of men being like women. The conditioning we have all received about what men should be is so deeply ingrained that many parents would baulk at allowing a son to go to nursery in pink socks, yet the sight of a little girl dressed in jeans riding a trike is perfectly acceptable. Images of women in charge are far more common than images of men caring for others.

Caring jobs are no less important than the others. Loving and nurturing should be part of the life of every human being – not just half of us. I do not believe that it is enough to encourage girls to do the things that boys have always done. Changes in the other direction are, if anything, more important. Nor is it enough to buy your son a doll. If Dad doesn't play with dolls, or care for babies, the chances are that son will not either. It looks as though boys will go on being boys until fathers take some responsibility for change.

DEVELOPMENTAL DIFFICULTIES

When to worry

If you are a real worrier you will read this first! Those calm and relaxed parents (who I envy so much) may never read it at all. What is in it is of no relevance at all to most parents because most of us will have children who do all the things discussed in these pages, in roughly the same order. If your child's development is nowhere near fitting into this general pattern this section may give you some guidance as to what you should do.

You know your child well. Your worries are not 'silly', even if they turn out to be unfounded. You have a right to ask for help. If there is something wrong your child will benefit from expert help at the earliest possible moment. If there is nothing wrong, you may well benefit from having someone with whom to discuss your worries and help you get them into proportion. There is absolutely no need to fear that a child referred for tests or special assistance will be unfairly labelled. A secondary school in Hackney (London) urges in its school booklet 'be an interfering parent'. It is a slogan we can all hang on to. Our children need us to interfere on their behalf.

Regular monitoring should be offered at your local baby clinic so that your baby's progress can be assessed. In the early months monitoring will be mainly of height and weight. Developmental testing is usually carried out by health visitors at around ten months, eighteen months, two and a half and four and a half years. However, you can ask for assessment at any time if you are worried. If you have specific concerns you should say so. Your information may provide vital clues to something which could otherwise be totally overlooked.

General development

Babies are not passive, floppy creatures. They may sleep a great deal and some are very calm between sleeps, gazing at their own hands waving, or listening to sounds. Even a calm baby should be responsive and turn towards interesting sounds, stare at a face, or cry if feeds are too long delayed. If your baby seems floppy and unresponsive, and does not become more muscular and alert over the first couple of months, you would be wise to talk to your doctor as there may be something holding him back. You can expect your child to move on from one stage to the next more or less as I have described in this chapter. If your child is lagging behind you will lose nothing by asking your Health Visitor, or doctor, to take a look.

Hearing and speech

These are closely related. A child who cannot hear will not learn to speak without help. A baby who can hear will turn towards sounds that are interesting – the sound of paper being crinkled, the doorbell ringing, a voice calling from another room. Towards the end of the first year the baby will start to imitate sounds. If he is showing no signs of forming words at two and no sign of stringing them together at two and a half it is in your child's best interests to ask for tests. Some children do not start speaking until they are three (or even four in rare cases), so there may be nothing wrong at all, but if there is a problem you will be giving him the best possible chance of learning to communicate effectively as soon as possible. An unnoticed problem could severely hamper your child when he starts school. If there is nothing wrong you can stop worrying.

Hearing difficulties may be present at birth or they may develop in infancy. All children should have their hearing tested by the end of the first year and all children who suffer from ear infections should be regularly tested in early childhood. Many hearing problems can be treated. Unfortunately testing is often carried out in inappropriate conditions by inexpert staff so that many problems (even severe ones) may go unnoticed.

It helps to be aware of how hard it is to test for hearing loss. A deaf child will very soon learn to use all her other senses to fill in the hearing gap. She will be keyed up to pick up any communication, however subtle. She will respond to guidance from you in the form of facial expression, movement and slight vibration. She may whirl round when a door slams – it may be the only noise she can hear. She may be able to follow simple instructions by lip reading and respond to music because she can feel the beat. She may well be able to hear low sounds (car noises, even aeroplanes) but miss all the high-pitched ones.

If your child 'passes' a routine hearing test and yet you are still not convinced that all is well, ask for a referral to a specialist department for more accurate tests. Be firm. In Nottingham, where parents have been given direct access to a specialist unit (without having to wait for referral from a GP or Health Visitor), most were found to have been correct about their worries.

Speech problems are not always related to hearing. The problem may be quite simple: perhaps a second child was born just as your child was learning to talk and the shock has set him back a bit. Time, patience and love will sort out this problem. A child who spends most of the day with a dummy in her mouth may also have difficulties. It may help to try cutting down the amount of time she uses it. Maybe you could have dummy times just before sleep.

Some children just do not hear enough speech to get the opportunity to learn, as this mother discovered:

> 'A friend of mine took her little boy aged two-and-a-half to a clinic because he never said a word. They asked if she talked to him. "No," she said. "How else will he learn"? they said. My boy was one year old at the time. I haven't stopped talking to him since. I tell him everything I'm doing, describing my actions in detail. At two-and-a-half he has a very good vocabulary.'

Children don't learn primarily from other children. They need to be talked to, often, by adults who are close to them and tuned in enough to pick up their cues and help them build up their language. If your child spends most of the day with other adults you need to make sure that they are taking on this rôle. If you fear your child is not being talked to enough, try to discuss this with your child carer. Make sure that you don't lose any opportunities yourself. Talk at breakfast time, bath time and bedtime, and give your child plenty of time to talk back. If this is not helping, ask for your child to be professionally assessed.

Children who have two languages to learn may take a little longer to get started, though this is not always the case. Paula and her husband speak Portuguese and Polish at home and their children speak English at school. She says:

> 'Our first boy did not start speaking until his second birthday. I put it down to the fact that he was being brought up with two languages but I don't think it had anything to do with it. Our second boy started speaking when he was just over one year old and he could produce correct sentences in both languages. For those parents who hesitate about bringing their children up with a foreign language – don't. For children it's as simple as breathing. My older two have no problems with English – no problems with reading or writing. They started

*nursery with just the bare essentials. After just a few weeks they were
quite competent.'*

Eyes

As soon as your baby can move her head she should start responding to what
she can see – a light source, faces moving across her cot. As her vision
adjusts, she will gaze at mobiles, leaves waving in the wind and anything
which catches her attention. Often vision and sound will come together: she
will move to look at your face because she can hear your voice. However, in
a quiet room she should also look up when you turn on a light, look towards
the window when the curtain opens and, in time, return a smile with a smile
of her own. Your child's sight will automatically be tested at the clinic but
if she does not seem to be responding to visual stimuli, you should mention
it.

Something else you may notice at this early stage is a squint, or lazy
eye. A squint needs to be identified and treated as soon as possible. Without
treatment, one eye will be used less and less until eventually sight in that
eye may be lost altogether. In the first few months many children look as
though they squint. By the fourth month a true squint is easier to identify.
One eye follows you around the room, the other does not. Early treatment
involves covering the better eye in order to encourage vision in the other
one. Surgery may also be suggested at a later stage.

As your child starts to play, to reach out to objects, and finally to try to
read, you may become aware that, although he can see, his vision is impaired.
If he is long-sighted he may have difficulty playing with small objects close
to him. He may prefer to talk to you from a distance rather than sitting on
your knee, and you might find him backing away in order to look at things.

A short-sighted child may be harder to spot at first. Ball games may be
difficult (he cannot see the ball until it has hit him) and he may prefer
small-scale activities. Sitting close to the television is probably not a good
indication (many children with perfectly good sight seem to practically climb
inside the set). If you suspect short sight you can make a rough check by
getting him to identify distant pictures or objects. My short sight was discovered when I couldn't see a flag flying on top of a building.

A child who cannot see adequately will have to make an enormous extra
effort to do the things that she wants to do. Whole areas of activity may be
virtually impossible and severe short sight can be positively dangerous. Your
child's sight will be checked for major problems at developmental tests but
less severe problems are unlikely to show up. If you suspect a problem, it is
best to get a thorough test from an optician or opthalmologist. Glasses will
not make your child's eyes improve but they will improve his vision. Point
out to him that looking at pictures or doing puzzles is easier if you can see

and, as long as he is comfortable, he will probably find it a wonderful improvement. However, there is no need to insist on your child wearing glasses all the time, if he is happier, though hazier without them.

Behavioural problems

There are no ways of measuring behaviour. Some children seem to be able to play calmly and quietly for hours – others need constant attention and will demand it loudly if they are not getting it. Some develop habits which they find soothing, perhaps rocking themselves to sleep or hair-twiddling, or becoming totally devoted to a cloth or soft toy – others don't. The range of what is perfectly normal is vast. You should expect your child to go through difficult periods (see Chapter 3) but sometimes children seem to get stuck in a difficult phase for longer than you can cope with or start behaving in a way which you consider odd.

   The hardest part is to try and stand back so that you can see your own child objectively. What seems odd close up may not seem so from a safe distance. Talking to friends could help. Mostly they will try to reassure you but if you make it clear that you are really worried a friend may help you to decide whether you need help or whether you have the whole thing out of proportion.

> 'I thought I knew what children were like. Then I had a third and found that I had just been lucky with the first two. I assumed that if you say "do this" they would do it. This child just said "no". I was visiting a friend and he started hitting her child. I suddenly felt – there is something wrong. I was completely isolated. I didn't know whether this was a phase he would come through or a behavioural problem. There is no one to tell you "don't worry, this often happens." '

It helps to choose your confidante with care. The mother of a couple of little angels who never scream and kick may consider abnormal any behaviour out of the range that she is used to. The best support will come from someone who has 'been there'. Just talking about it and hearing someone else's reaction will be a terrific relief. If you are still worried, ask your doctor about a referral to your local Child Guidance Clinic.

OUR FEELINGS ABOUT PROBLEMS

If you discover that your child does have a problem it is your own feelings that you have to confront first. The difficulties your child is facing are, as yet, unchanged. Your initial feeling will probably be a mixture of fear and grief. Kathy Robinson, in her book *Children of Silence* (Gollancz, 1987), talks about how she felt when she discovered that her daughter was deaf:

> 'There were only two stages in my life now: before knowing about Sarah's deafness and after. Did Mr Chapman realise what his words had done? They had changed our lives for ever. Before we were an ordinary family. Now deafness had come to set us apart and make us different. We were on our own. Alone.'

People with disabilities often tell us that their biggest problem is coping with the attitudes of able-bodied people. A child who is born with a disability of some kind, or acquires it soon after birth, is already 'coping' with her disability as well as she is able. She is used to being the way she already is. It is we who have to get used to the situation. The way we approach it will shape the way our children are. Isabel had a baby with a hare lip. She describes a visit to the hospital with her baby:

> 'One of the first things we learned was that children are what their parents are. We saw two children with an illness which made them look strange. Their eyes bulged and there were scars on their cheeks. One child was chattering away with everyone in the most friendly way. The other looked oppressed and sad and sick. We looked at their mothers and it was staggering. The mother of the first boy was speaking to another woman, incredibly alive and amused. The mother of the second boy looked so tense that I was waiting almost to see her starting to scream in a fit. She looked ashamed and asking for forgiveness for having a child like that.'

We are our children's first mirrors of the way they will be in the world. We have to come to terms with the way they are and not to crave for them to be the way we want them. Says Isabel:

> 'I tried from the beginning to be very natural with George. He saw the pictures we took and we talked a lot about it. Not long ago I saw him with a mirror looking intently at his face. I asked why he was looking in the mirror. "My lip," said George. "Why?" I asked. "Do you know Mum I have found that I can whistle without anyone noticing it. I do tricks at school," he said. I felt wonderful because he has such a positive attitude.'

Self confidence grows out of other people's respect, not out of their pity. We need to learn to respect our children and then to demand respect from them from the people around us. But first we need to accept ourselves and our own feelings. Covering up our inevitable feelings of grief, guilt and anger will not help us to accept our children as they are. Parents of children with disabilities have the same need as all parents to find others with whom they can share their anxieties and express their fears. Sadly the attitudes of able-bodied people may be hostile or uncomprehending. Says Isabel:

> *'English middle-class people didn't seem to see anything. As though nothing was wrong when George had an enormous gap in his mouth. I felt that black, Latino and working-class people were infinitely more natural and more healthy. They would ask me about it which meant I could explain everything and that was a tremendous relief.'*

Sharing and support

Just as a parent of a crying baby gets most help from other parents going through the same experience, parents of children with disabilities may well find it helpful to share their feelings openly with people who have had to come to terms with similar experiences. Having a child who needs special attention may put an enormous strain on other children in the family and on relationships with partners. You may need help in fighting to get the best possible treatment or special equipment for your child.

While you and your child have every right to make use of all the existing facilities for children (indeed you will probably find the children a great deal more accepting than their parents), it will probably help if you also make contact with organisations established to support people with disabilities. Many have parents' support groups. Your health visitor may well be able to put you in touch. If you want more help with dealing with your feelings than you feel you can get from other parents, you might want to consider individual or family therapy. The Women's Therapy Centre (see p. 210) have run group therapy sessions for mothers of children with disabilities and they may be able to put you in touch with a similar group or with an individual therapist.

Chapter 3

SETTING LIMITS

I never did, I never did, I never *did* like 'Now take care, dear!'
I never did, I never did, I never *did* want 'Hold my hand;'
I never did, I never did, I never *did* think much of 'Not up there, dear!'
It's no good saying it. They don't understand.

(A. A. Milne, When We Were Very Young)

WHO NEEDS LIMITS?

'Children need to know the limits – it is an essential part of their security – of knowing that a parent is encircling their world with a perimeter. Within this perimeter they can act with confidence and assurance. They constantly push at the perimeter and the parent's role is to redefine the limits as the child's self-confidence and skills increase.'

At first we applaud every move forward our children make – smiling, holding, sitting, walking – then at some stage we start to say no. At first it is usually just a matter of safety.

'I take the view that, at eleven months, a baby only needs to know the word "no" about things that are dangerous: such as touching the stove, falling down stairs and pulling the video on her head.'

As they grow and start to strive for independence we have to make daily compromises between our children's safety and their search for independence.

'My daughter simply refuses to hold my hand in the street. At two and a half she likes to strut along at least a couple of yards away, swinging her bag and gazing in shop windows. "Are you pretending to be on your own?" I asked, and she grinned. So I agreed to compromise. She can walk on her own as long as she stays close to me and promises to hold my hand when crossing roads.'

In a city the desire to mix with other children holds special dangers.

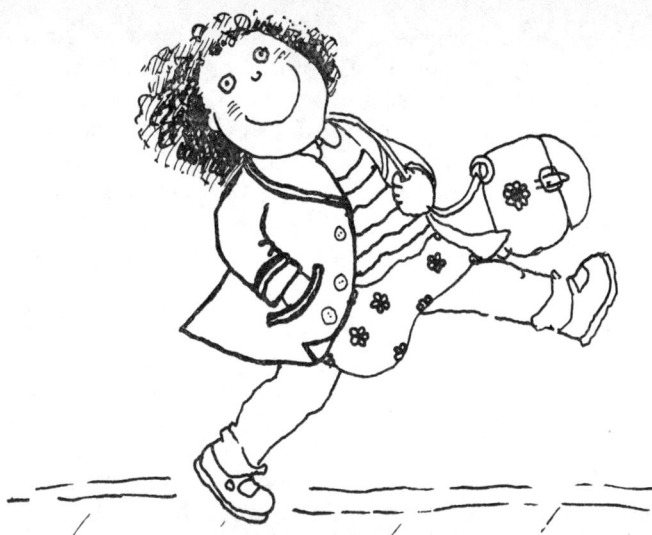

'Mick desperately wants to play out with the other kids. At three years old I really don't feel I can trust him not to run into the street after a ball. So I keep him in and he hates me for it.'

Protecting ourselves

We set limits not only to protect our children but also to protect ourselves. Just as we have to consider their needs for exploration, food, sleep and attention when we arrange our lives, they also have to learn to consider our needs. They have to learn that we are not multi-handed, computer-operated, loving providers of their every desire.

'Demanding attention as soon as the telephone rings went on for a long time. I know why, but it was always difficult to cope with. At best I would make a fuss of them as soon as the call was over. They weren't, as I saw it, behaving badly, only naturally – and very consistently.'

Some parents feel the need to start setting limits in the first few months just to get some space for themselves if, for example, their children's sleeping or feeding patterns have become intolerable. (These issues are discussed in Chapters 4 and 5.) While it is certainly possible to *train* children to perform in certain ways, this kind of behaviour-shaping will not teach the kind of self discipline and thoughtfulness which will provide the basis for decisions and judgements in later life. While it may be necessary at certain times its value for a child's development is extremely limited.

Helping our children to learn the value of being considerate with us helps them to learn ways of co-existing with other people. As social beings, they will spend the rest of their lives using, and improving on, these skills. What they learn in these early years they will take with them into relationships in their wider world. For some children these lessons are very easy to learn. Others seem to be so completely absorbed in the struggle for freedom and independence that the value of cooperation takes a great deal longer to learn.

DRAWING OUR OWN LINE

Good and bad behaviour is not a fixed goal. It is something that we parents establish for ourselves, taking into account our own needs and the social circle in which we live. Every society and every family has some rules. Some insist that children should be polite to older people but are very relaxed about bedtime. Others encourage their children to question authority and consider a certain amount of 'backchat' amusing but are absolutely adamant about regular bedtimes. You make your own rules. If you want to live harmoniously with your children they will have to learn what is important to you. The clearer and more consistent you can be, the more easily they will learn.

'I would like the children to learn to keep their rooms tidy and to do a small share of housework as soon as they are able. Unfortunately they need only look at my room and they can say, quite legitimately, "Why don't you tidy your own room first?". I know I will never get anywhere until I can practise what I preach.'

As a bottom line most people would agree that 'children must learn to consider other people and their feelings.' Most parents would formulate additional goals as their children get older:

'I want Raoul to finish what he starts. To be aware of how difficult it is to keep a house in order (for example by taking care of his clothes and toys), and to realise that, without effort, we cannot do anything.'

It is a fortunate parent who finds the job of providing those limits as effortless as this mother of a three-year-old:

'I find the idea of discipline completely inappropriate to a very small child. Rosa is never punished. I have always tried to negotiate with her. She behaves very well in public, trying to pick up what is expected of her. I am only interested in developing what is in her, not in imposing rules.'

If, on reading that, you feel like spitting, the probability is you are the lucky parent of a child who never stops pushing at the limits of safety, your patience and his or her own physical abilities.

'Jo was very aggressive. He would run around the playgroup pushing other children and throwing toys. I always felt very defensive about his behaviour. I tried the tone-of-voice ploy but that never worked. The sitting on a chair in a quiet corner didn't work either. He never seemed to object to being told off, but neither did he listen or take any notice of what I said. I have ended up shouting and smacking and I hate myself for it as in my heart I believe that it just perpetuates and perhaps reinforces bad behaviour, but, after so much, my temper snaps.'

or

'Rob has never learned to play quietly by himself. He wants my attention absolutely all the time and, if he doesn't get it, he will deliberately do something naughty in order to get it. If I have a friend here he will be jumping all over them, climbing on the table, making as much noise as possible – anything to ensure that he is not excluded. Going out with him is a nightmare.'

Helping your child to become a happy, fulfilled, and cooperative member of society can be as worrying and upsetting as it is exciting and fulfilling. But Jo's mother, now her son has turned five, can say of him:

'He is happy and eager to learn, still a bit loud and silly, but no longer a disruptive element in class. He joins in everything and is open to everything and has lots of friends and I love him and like him very much.'

What is it that makes one child cooperative and easy-going and another one difficult and unmanageable? Of course, at either end of the spectrum there are children who have been cowed into submission or turned into little monsters by totally inappropriate treatment. A child who is locked in a cupboard, beaten, or otherwise abused is unlikely to behave 'normally'. However, in between these extremes lies a vast range of behaviour from aggression and disobedience to shyness and clinginess. For every parent who worries about his child's unmanageable behaviour there will be another who is concerned about her child's anxiety.

Children are different. One child bursts into tears if an unfamiliar adult speaks slightly sharply to him, another doesn't seem to register until you are holding on to him and making your feelings known very clearly. The first child has absorbed his own limits and only needs the most gentle reinforcement, the second child seems to need constant, firm guidance and will probably take a great deal longer to learn how to function in society without creating waves.

This second child may be hard to live with but (if he is not too heavily sat upon) may retain his desire to push at the limits and explore and challenge as he grows up. The first child will probably learn quite early the value of cooperation which will enhance not only his own life but the lives of those around him. Both kinds of behaviour are valid and both kinds of children could learn plenty of value from each other. The timid child may grow up happier if he learns the value of assertiveness. The pushy child could learn a lot about responsiveness. But nothing we do as parents will make these children the same.

The fact that children are so different makes it hard for us to sort out what is in our heads and what is in theirs; whether we are over-reacting or not intervening enough; whether we are facing a real problem or a passing phase. We need to share strategies for living through the difficult times, and help our children to draw useful lessons from them.

FINDING A STRATEGY

The power of being positive

Young children are not altruistic. They want to do what makes them happy. The thing is to let them know that you share the same goals. They are more likely to be pleasant to others if they discover that this gives them greater pleasure than knocking them over and pinching their toys. Their behaviour will be reinforced if they can see, by our example, that they get more, and better quality, attention from being pleasant than from biting and hitting us.

There is usually a way of getting our children to cooperate because they want to, not just because we want them to.

'Rosa would never get out of the bath. I started warming the towel on a radiator and then I would hold it up for her to get into. She loved the feeling of being parcelled up in the warmth. If she dallied getting out I would comment on how the towel was getting cooler and, if she didn't hurry it would soon be cold. She loved the whole ritual and rarely complained about getting out.'

Explaining, distracting, turning a difficult journey into a game does take time. Sometimes it seems to be extra time that we haven't got, or it involves creative thinking that we are too tired or harrassed to exercise, but if we can find ways of making the time it pays dividends:

'The ten-minute walk to nursery used to take up to half an hour whatever I did. If I was feeling short-tempered I would simply spend the time snapping and telling him to hurry up. Then I would often end up carrying him to stop him running off in the opposite direction. On

good days we would play games: find me a red car, let's count the cats in the gardens. I chose games which would make him run eagerly, and happily, in the right direction.'

Between three and five years old children are particularly keen to start taking control of their own world. Explanation will work far better than instruction at this stage and the more scope you give for independent action the more cooperative your child is likely to be. She needs to know that what she is doing is her own idea.

'When children were grabbing things off supermarket shelves I would say "Don't take those things, we don't need them. Help me find the things we do want – can you find the beans?" etc. If I had time I would also talk about the things they had grabbed – "They are nice shapes, colours and so on," while putting them back. If they still went on with it I would stop them more firmly.'

A confrontation avoided is far better than a battle won. Sometimes we need to find strategies which allow our children to 'climb down' without losing dignity. If your child simply refuses to do something you ask it may be that he just feels driven into a corner. It can help simply to change the subject: 'Look! Did you see that bird over there? What beautiful feathers it's got . . .'.

'When we reached deadlock I could feel the anger squeezing through mixed up with a sort of desperation. When he was between two and four years old I developed a game which seemed to work every time. I would stand very still and say "shut your eyes." Then I would say very calmly; "I think there is another little boy in there who really wants to be good. Why don't you ask him to come out and play with me?" He always entered into the spirit of it and, usually with obvious relief he would be wonderfully cooperative . . . until the next time.'

However tired or rushed you feel it is still worth trying to find that extra ounce of energy if only because doing something happily with your children will make you feel happy too.

We cannot always manage to handle our children as we would like, though it is worth remembering that our children model their behaviour on ours. They do not like our bad temper any more than we like theirs, but they will learn from it. If we shout and order them about they are learning that the way to get what you want is to shout and order people about. As one parent commented:

'Someone I know hits her child when he is aggressive. It makes him worse – what does she expect?'

This is not to say that every moment of anger is being recorded in some future store of knowledge, or that our every bad mood moves one more step towards the creation of a delinquent. Our children are separate beings who must eventually take responsibility for their own lives. We can help them if we demonstrate the value of negotiation over confrontation, the use of words rather than fists, and the value of being able to apologise when we know we are in the wrong.

Firmer lines

For some parents life is a daily struggle to establish even the most general baseline of what is acceptable: to prevent their children doing things that are dangerous to themselves and others.

'At the age of two, Jo seemed to be unable to sit down and play. His idea of a good time was to run around the room pushing the other children over and disturbing their activities.'

From my own observation of a group of young children in a crêche as well as my experience of my own and friends' children I think that most have gone through patches of behaving in a way which was fairly alarming to their parents. Periods of aggression with other children and obstinate refusal to cooperate with adults usually cause the most concern.

We had children who would bite and scratch if they didn't get their way, and fight over toys. All of them came out of these periods of antisocial behaviour and have clearly learned from them. Some passed through in a matter of weeks, others took much longer, and most tended to return to these difficult behaviour patterns in times of stress.

Avoidable and Unavoidable stress

Sometimes children are reacting to stress which they cannot understand or explain. We have to try and work it out for them and, if possible, do something to relieve it.

Lack of safe space
Young children need space to run and explore without being constantly told off. Lack of safe space is probably one of the most important contributors to difficult behaviour. A report on children in bed and breakfast hotels (*A Prescription for Poor Health* by the London Food Commission, Maternity Alliance, Shelter and SHAC, The London Housing Aid Centre, 1988) found:

'Nearly a quarter were identified as being unusually aggressive or active. Many mothers felt their children's behaviour had deteriorated and they had become "wild", "cheeky", or "out of control".'

As one of the mothers interviewed in the report said:

> 'They seemed very tense and aware of the situation, leading to
> naughtiness, tantrums and screaming. I can't tell them to go to
> another room. You just have to put up with it somehow.'

Parents and children in bed and breakfast are at a special disadvantage
when trying to sort out a way of being together. However, space constraints
are not confined to homeless people.

> 'I was pregnant with twins and had recently moved into our home and
> we were taking it apart. So life at home was pretty grim.'

> 'We moved when he was eighteen months and lived with some very un-
> child-oriented people. His freedom was very limited. We had no
> outside play space, our personal space was extremely restricted and
> there were stair gates to keep him out of their space. The kitchen was
> not child-proof so I had to watch him all the time. I was even told off
> for letting him play with the pots and pans. Thank God he had more
> freedom with his childminder.'

Lack of attention

Children also need attention and, if they do not get it, they will react with
either anger or sadness. Most studies of child development have concluded
that it is the quality of the attention we give that is important, not the
quantity. It is perfectly possible to spend hours with children without giving
them any attention at all.

> 'In the park the other day I noticed a woman with two children of about
> eighteen months and three years old. We were there for over and hour
> and, while the children played in the sand, she read a book. Her only
> contact with them was, occasionally, to stop the younger one from
> climbing out.'

On the other hand you can work all day and be so looking forward to seeing
your children that you give them all your attention during the period you
are together. This teenage mother was interviewed by Sue Sharpe in her
book *Falling for Love*, after she returned to college:

> 'I love them now, I don't really think I loved them before, I was too
> bored by it all, I think, too depressed. Now I spend less time with
> them, I really enjoy them.'

When we are depressed, over-worked, or coping with difficulties in relationships, it's hard to give children real attention, to let them know that we
enjoy them. It's at times like this that our children are most likely to add
to the pressure we are under by the way they behave. Yinka was just over

two. He had a new baby brother and his mother had just returned to a stressful full-time job.

> 'He went through a very difficult patch. He refused to join games. He would fly into fits of crying if anyone tried to discipline him and he was extremely aggressive to his younger brother. His behaviour improved dramatically when his father took to spending a couple of hours alone with him every afternoon.'

The birth of a sibling can trigger or contribute to problems of aggression, as Sandra discovered:

> 'Graham used to stand behind me on the settee and try to strangle me as I fed his sister. How she survived I don't know.'

Relieving stress

These situations have many common strands. They describe circumstances in which a child has been frustrated by too little space, too many limits on behaviour and a sudden loss of attention. If we can work out what is troubling our children we can sometimes find strategies for relieving the stress.

Making more physical space is one of the hardest problems, but it does help to pack away breakable objects and make your home as safe as possible so that you do not have to keep saying no. You can also check out all the available childcare facilities and children's play amenities (see Chapter 7).

Making time may be easier but you may have to neglect something else in order to provide it. Cathy ran into problems with her third child after working full time, without any problems, with the first two:

> 'He was three and a half and his behaviour had got completely out of hand. He was unhappy and aggressive and I was miserable and guilty. One night as I was putting him to bed he said: "Mummy, you make me feel so sad and cross." I felt that I had failed as a mother and I worked myself into a right state. Finally, feeling very disloyal to my son, I went to my boss and said: "My youngest child is having behavioural problems. I need to take time off." It was so hard to do it and yet, I only needed to ask. I am not the only one who takes time off and makes it up on other days. It made a significant difference and it was an enormous relief to be able to look back and say "There was a problem, I wasn't imagining it." Tackling it made all the difference.'

If our attention is taken up by problems in our own relationships or by our own unhappiness it is hard to find the energy to be really 'with' our children. Our children want us to *enjoy* them and to do that we need to be feeling open to them and reasonably happy with ourselves. Sometimes we find that the best way to make our children happy and cooperative is to take time making ourselves happy.

> *'Time spent on me is not time taken away from my children. The better I feel the better the time we spend together and the happier we all are.'*

Couples going to child guidance sessions often find that the guidance is not needed for their children but for themselves. Sessions may lead to sorting out problems in their own relationship and finding ways of dealing with stress which does not mean dumping it on their children.

Single parents may have less of this kind of stress. The lines of authority are clearer, as one recently separated mother said:

> *'Separating has been the best thing that has happened to me since I became a mother. I no longer have to negotiate about who is getting Paul up in the morning. I just do it.'*

Nevertheless, parents who are on their own (and many women in couples are essentially on their own) can run into different kinds of difficulties. It is hard not to have someone with an equal stake in a child's future with whom you can discuss things. Your own feelings of insecurity may prevent you from being calm and make your children feel insecure too. Finding someone outside the situation who can act as a sounding-board for your fears may help you to come to terms with your feelings. As you gain confidence in your own ability to be a parent, your children will gain confidence in you. (See 'How we can help each other', pp. 57–63.)

HOW WE FEEL

We have to find ways of dealing with our own feelings too. Few of us are so saintly that we are actually patient and easy-going all the time. Indeed, it is probably important that our children know that we can be angry, and that we will still go on loving them afterwards. Sometimes children go on and on pushing in an apparent attempt to make us lose control. Perhaps that is exactly what they are doing: trying to find out where our patience stops. Maybe they need to find out that it is all right to express anger sometimes rather than bottling it all up.

On really bad days the feeling of being 'out of control' can be overwhelming. We feel that we are hopeless parents and that our children will grow up to be delinquents. Sometimes we forget that our children are probably not enjoying these phases very much either. We all need a break. At these times it helps to try and carve out small islands of peace where you and your child can remind each other that you are loved and that you care for each other.

It may help to find something to do together which could not possibly result in a mess all over the floor and you in a rage and does not demand anything (even a thank you) in return from your child. Reading stories is pretty safe and a good time to be physically close, or you could take time out to sit and watch children's television with your child on your knee. Something as simple as arranging a meal in the shape of a face on the plate and then eating together can be a gesture which will remind you that you love one another in spite of the difficulties.

It is when your child is at her most difficult that it is most important to remember that praise is more powerful than blame. Showing pleasure when your child actually gets into the bath without a fuss will have more effect on her behaviour than your anger when you have to endure a battle.

Many mothers suffer from Pre Menstrual Syndrome (PMS), which makes the days before a period very hard to cope with. We may feel tired and snappy and find it almost impossible to produce that extra ounce of energy which may avert a crisis:

'I know he doesn't like cold chicken so I had fried it with vegetables. It had taken time to do. When he pushed it away and said "I'm not hungry," I just went crazy and shouted at him to leave the room. I know I was being irrational. I felt I had no control left.'

Mealtimes are often the trigger for some of our most irrational behaviour.

'I felt so irritable and cross that just the sight of him eating spaghetti with his mouth open gave me an almost insurmountable urge to push his face into the plate. I resisted it but a friend I confessed to related the story of her mother doing precisely what had been going through my mind. Apparently her brother had been stirring up his shepherd's pie into a grey mush and, overcome with rage, she picked up the plate and emptied the whole lot over his head. I expect the job of cleaning up afterwards undid any satisfaction she may have got from the gesture.'

Of course most of us, most of the time, do not act on these feelings. We push them down and bottle them up, but it helps to release that tension – not by tipping food over our children but by talking to other parents about our bad moments and finding ways to turn tension into laughter. If you know the time you are most likely to feel bad it helps to try and plan ahead. Try to avoid situations which are likely to be stressful and arrange for friends and other family members to help out at those times. Perhaps you could arrange a swop with a friend who also has PMS . . . at a different time of the month. Or arrange for another child to visit, which can take the intensity out of the situation and give your child someone else to focus on.

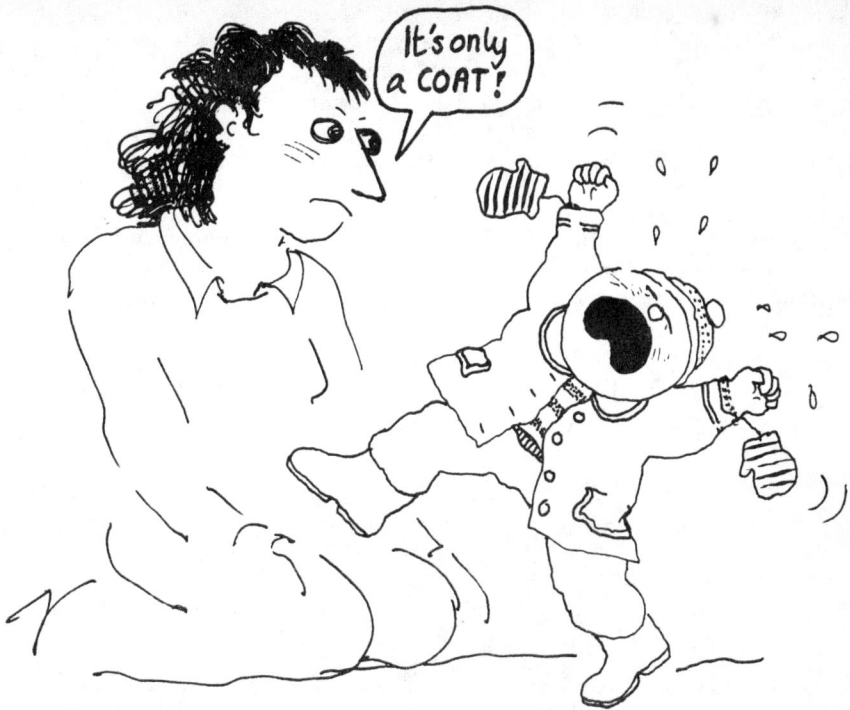

TIME TO SAY NO

Even if we have sorted out any underlying problems affecting our children's behaviour there will still be times when cooperation, attention, and a firm 'no' are simply not enough. Then we have to deal with the issue of discipline – just how to go about making it clear to our children that we are in control.

There are times when a firm 'no', with a brief explanation, is the best approach. On occasions too much explanation may be misunderstood and actually add to the problem.

> 'When Rosa went through a phase of scratching we would make her apologise to the child and then "kiss and make up". She really enjoyed the apologising and kissing but would then go on five minutes later to scratch someone else. It occurred to me that she may be doing the scratching in order to get the kissing and the praise for being a good girl. So we stopped asking her to apologise and just told her firmly that scratching was bad. She stopped doing it pretty quickly.'

It takes time for children to learn what is acceptable to us and we need to keep repeating the lessons.

'*Daytime public exhibitions I try to ignore as best I can and just
continue with what has to be done, i.e. putting on a coat, even if it
means having a child pinned over my knee screaming blue murder. I
try very hard not to get cross but I don't give in either as I feel quite
strongly that they have to accept certain limits and restrictions and
that, as long as these remain constant, they can only be to their benefit
in the long term.*'

If we keep the 'nos' to the minimum necessary for harmonious living we
stand a better chance of success, but it is important to be consistent about
the things that really matter. This is probably particularly important if you
have a very rebellious child who seems to take advantage of every momentary lapse in attention. If Johnny is not allowed to help himself to food most
of the time, but allowed to eat all the fruit in the bowl at those times when
you happen to be distracted by a phonecall, he is getting a very mixed
message. Better to keep the bowl out of reach than to descend vengefully
when he has already rubbed the grapes into the carpet.

When 'no' is not enough

This is the mother of a child of eighteen months:

'*So far I really do hope I never physically punish my child. I find it
really difficult to know what to say when I see other adults doing it
– it is shocking to see the level of uninhibited violence against quite
small toddlers that happens so much in this country.*'

On the other hand some parents see smacking as a necessary reinforcement
of discipline. Says one:

'*If he was spitting, or kicking, I wouldn't just say "Oh he doesn't
understand." I would restrain him, or take him away or smack his
legs. I did it to establish who was in charge.*'

However she was aware that:

'*If you do smack you have to be very careful it doesn't get out of hand.*'

The regular use of smacking (occasionally and lightly – not beating) as a
form of discipline seems to have more to do with class and culture than
degrees of love for children. An occasional smack is probably less damaging
than long periods of angry silence. However, child psychiatrist and grand-
father Bruno Bettelheim, in his book *A Good Enough Parent* (Thames and
Hudson, 1987), has this to say:

'*While criticism or fear of punishment may restrain us from doing
wrong, it does not make us wish to do right. Disregarding this simple*

fact is the great error into which parents and educators fall when they rely on these negative means of correction. The only effective discipline is self discipline, motivated by the inner desire to feel good about oneself – "have a good conscience". It is not much of a conscience which tells us not to do wrong because we might get punished. The effective conscience motivates us to do right because we know that otherwise we will suffer all the pain and depression of feeling bad about ourselves.'

That is all very well, but many parents who fundamentally agree with this philosophy guiltily admit to 'snapping and smacking'. They would probably also admit that it doesn't do much to stop the bad behaviour. 'He just goes off and does the same thing five minutes later.'

It is clearly illogical to try and teach a child not to be aggressive by using aggression. We must find ways of dealing with our own anger. Our children are perfectly capable of maddening us beyond reason. We need to find ways of coping with them which will help us regain control and let them know that they have gone right over the bounds of what is reasonable.

'When I am angry I often chuck him out of the room – he hates that, so he realises his misbehaviour was serious and it gets him out of the way so that I don't get any angrier.'

'I would make her sit on the stairs. It frankly amazed me that she would do it. She would be crying her eyes out and yelling with fury but she wouldn't move until I told her too. Then she would usually be very contrite.'

Bettelheim agrees that the best way to let a child know when he or she has done wrong is:

'to ban the child, for a short while from our presence. We may send him out of the room, or, if possible, to his own room. Or we may withdraw to our own room.'

He reasons that the best sanction is one that induces the child to 'correct his behaviour, now and in the future for *his* reasons, and not for the reasons of the parent.' He suggests that since a parent's love is something every child needs, the threat of losing that love, even for a moment, is the most effective deterrent.

HOW WE CAN HELP EACH OTHER

Other carers

Consistent limits are far easier to maintain if all the people caring for a child have the same views and enforce them in much the same way. Children

I couldn't help it,....he would've had a tantrum....

SWEETiES!

Pops

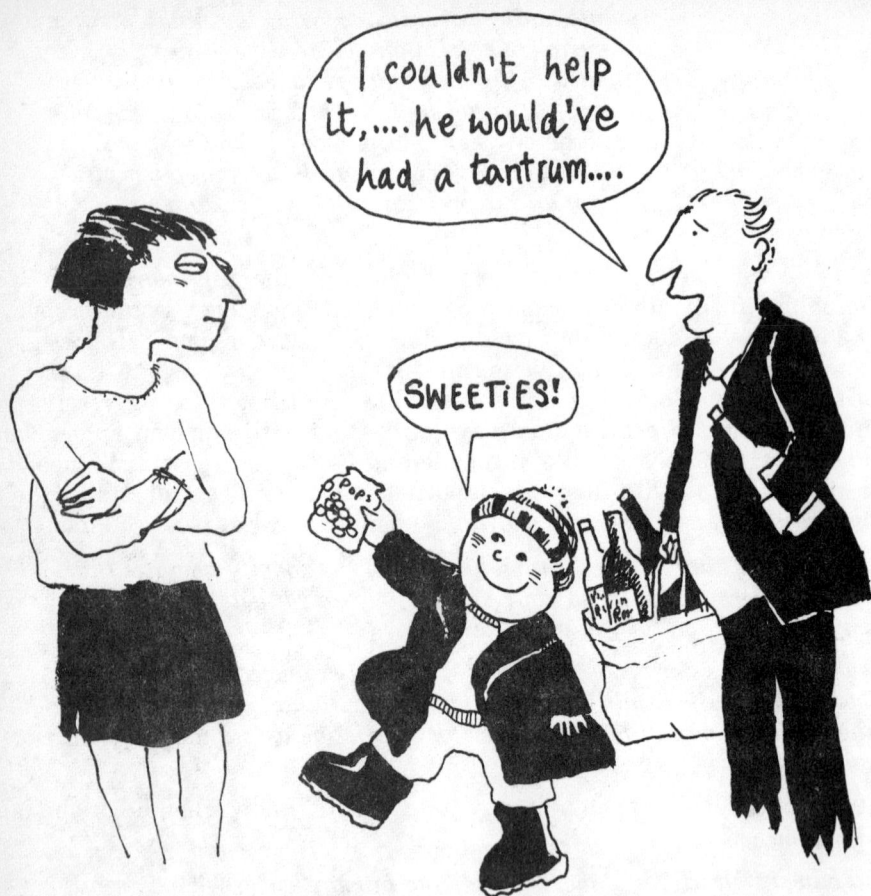

can cope with some difference between nursery and home. The problems arise when two different people are imposing two sets of values in the same space and at the same time. In an extended family the tension can arise between grandparents and parents. Most often it arises between partners and, given a family structure in which most fathers are out of the house for longer hours than mothers, it is usually mothers who have to cope with the effects of differing policies. It is very frustrating to spend time with a child making a certain set of demands very clear and then find the whole lot undermined. Children very quickly realise that there is mileage to be made out of their parents' disagreements.

'I worry a lot about the children eating sweets and get angry with their father about it. He will go to the off-license with Jerome who will then come through the door saying "I'm going to tell Mummy I've got

some sweets," brandishing fruitgums. "I couldn't help it," his father
says. "He would have had a tantrum. He doesn't respect my authority
like he does yours." '

In fact this parent knows exactly why his partner does not give their children
sweets. He knows also that he is undermining her authority by buying them
and making her job a great deal more difficult. However, he enjoys being
able to be the person who provides treats and is not concerned about the
consequences because he will not have to cope with them. Such a difference
in approach is very undermining to a parent who is struggling to establish,
in this case, healthy eating patterns. It isn't helping the child either. He is
learning that he can manipulate his parents and, paradoxically, that will
probably make him feel insecure. After all, in most circumstances a child
wants the adults who care for him to be stronger and more reliable than he
is.

When there are two parents, establishing a clear, joint strategy is important and it seems reasonable that the parent who spends most of the time
with the children should take the lead in establishing such a policy. Yet
many fathers take on the rôle of family disciplinarian. Perhaps because they
have so little contact with their children, this gives them a spurious sense
of control. This can also undermine their partner's confidence.

*'My husband says I deal with it all wrong. He maintains that I just
waste my time keeping on and on to no effect. My opinion is that, if
I ask the kids to do something and they ignore me, if he's around he
should reinforce my request, not put me down in front of them.'*

Sometimes the end of a period of family tension is a new beginning for a
child.

*'When her father left, the tension in the house was reduced overnight.
She still behaved badly much of the time but I found that I could
usually reason with her, calmly and quietly. It was such a relief
knowing that her father was not going to storm in, and yell at her.'*

When parents act together they can provide each other with invaluable back-
up.

*'I work all day and sometimes at night. I am so tired that I do not feel
like putting on a lot of pressure but I am lucky because his father
takes his share of this.'*

Supporting each other

*'If my child behaves badly in public it makes me feel guilty. Specially
in England. In Spain there is much more patience with children.*

There seems to be an attitude that children are children and therefore unable sometimes to cope with reality. If a parent shouts at a child, people try to find excuses for the child. In England I feel that one is permanently under a sort of Inquisition that puts mothers on trial all the time. Society doesn't help mothers but at the same time demands constant perfection.'

We live in a society in which parents are held responsible for the deeds of their children and nobody accepts responsibility for anyone else's children. It is peculiar to the Anglo-Saxon way of life. Nowhere are children quite so uncared for at a social level. It is not just that we have hardly any nurseries in this country – it is embedded in our individual attitudes too. A playground superviser told me the following story:

'There was a woman in here the other day with two little children. She had the younger one, she was about eighteen months, in a swing and was twisting it round and then letting go so that it would spin around. I asked her to stop because it is dangerous and she said "these are my children and I will do what I like with them".'

The feeling that children are private possessions infects even people who are perfectly caring with their own children:

'The scene is a children's party. Parents and children are sitting around on the grass. Two children are playing in a sand pit and the older one (about three) decides to exert some power over the younger one (about eighteen months). First he hits her over the head with a spade, then he throws sand at her. The nearest adults look embarrassed, clearly waiting for someone to intervene, but the parents of the aggressor are occupied elsewhere. In the end the younger child is lifted out screaming and its parents are heard to remark on the unfairness of life.'

Any of the adults could simply have intervened and either a) removed the spade or b) removed the older child, explaining quietly that such behaviour is not pleasant. However, to do so would have been tantamount to trespassing on someone else's property. Instead of quietly reprimanding the child (which would have been some help to the busy parents), a heavily charged atmosphere of disapproval grew around both him and his parents, who remained blissfully ignorant of their child's misdeeds.

An aggressive toddler is not a bad person. He or she has just not yet learned such social skills as negotiating or sharing. If we ignore this sort of behaviour we are not helping the struggle to find better ways of communicating. That doesn't mean we should over-react, or cut across a parent who is already dealing with the situation, but in the absence of a readily available parent or other carer quiet, firm guidance, even from a total stranger, can only add to a child's understanding of how to be a social being. This does not undermine or distract from a parent's authority – it can only support it. Indeed, a more genuinely concerned attitude to children might take some of the burden off the parents of an aggressive child. I know from my own experience how much harder it is to be the mother of the biter than the mother of the child who has been bitten:

> 'It is not just the distress of seeing your child inflict pain, it is the vengeance wreaked by other parents which really hurts. Some parents seem positively to gloat over their children's wounds: "Look what your Jill has done to my Jack. It's actually bleeding." Usually the child, responding to his parent's tone of voice, will start howling (or howling louder), revelling in the attention.'

Whose interests are served by this sort of performance? It makes the parents feel guilty and embarrassed. It may cause them to be unduly angry with their child in order to compensate. It probably encourages the bitten child to kick up a fuss over the slightest scrape in order to get all that attention and it makes the biter feel angry, confused and not at all sorry. How much better it would be for an adult to intervene straight away, explain why the behaviour is wrong, and leave it at that.

The tendency to blame individual parents for the behaviour of their children can lead people to assume that their own child must have 'caught' such behaviour from others. The mother of a fifteen-months-old boy says:

> 'He's never been shown aggressive behaviour by us but, since mixing with other children, he will push and scratch. I think children are naturally aggressive or passive. I don't like aggressive children therefore I just try to avoid them.'

It's an attitude which on a bigger scale can lead to difficulties like this:

> 'At two and a half he went to play group and he loved it. He was still very loud and silly but he was very interested and liked the workers and started to join in. Shortly after he joined he pushed a child down stairs just as her father was arriving to pick her up. He raised the roof and so it was decided to cut Jo's hours to "give the other children a rest from him". I was pregnant, our house was being taken apart and life was pretty grim. I felt very bitter that I was being penalised for his disruptive behaviour. As the workers explained to me, he wasn't naughty, he was just impossible to discipline.'

A disruptive child is a problem in a group and strategies have to be evolved for coping so that other children do not suffer. However, excluding a child of two and a half for bad behaviour is pretty extreme. In some cases it will lead to total withdrawal from all group situations. This means that the child's difficulties in socialising can only get more acute. If the behaviour has been caused by inappropriate discipline then forcing parents and child to spend more time together will again make things worse. If, as in Jo's case, it was partly his age, and partly a reaction to a lot of changes in his life, it will just make the period of adjustment harder for both of them to cope with. Fortunately Jo's mother reacted by getting professional advice from a Child Guidance clinic.

'My husband wasn't in favour but I persuaded him in the end and we had two sessions. The people we saw did not offer guidance as such. We talked about family relationships and they put a lot of emphasis on the fact that my son had a solid bedrock of love to rely on and it was obvious we were very close. After the second session they said they really didn't think there was a problem, just that some children cope with change and little traumas by withdrawing and some by being very loud: "Look at me, I am still here." '

Professional help gave this mother confidence in her ability to cope with Jo, but the real help came from the opportunity to get support from someone much closer:

'The main benefit came from my husband telling me how patient he thought I was. He had never told me that before.'

There are few societies in which mothers are left so alone with their children. As one mother said:

'Between three and four was the hardest time. She took so much energy. I was overwhelmed by her demands and her expectations. Children at that age simply cannot get all they need from one person.'

This mother had the help of grandparents and a nursery. Many of us have neither. We do not ask for help because our society has made a virtue out of the impossible. We cope in the most impossible circumstances (in a report on women in bed and breakfast, Conway, 1988), the incidence of non-accidental injury was found to be no higher than average in spite of the terrible living conditions). Yet if we feel too tired and drained to cope with our children's demands we feel that *we* have failed. But carers need to be cared for. We have a right to ask for support from our partners, families (if we have them) and from society, in the form of nurseries and other child-care facilities. While we are waiting for the changes, perhaps the best we can do is care more for each other.

'We hardly ever shout. It doesn't bother me if someone else tells Benny off. There is not sense of, how dare she, that's my job. That trust took a long time to build between us but, ever since the beginning I have always felt that whatever the problem I had with him, it could always get an airing.'

Carolyn was writing ('Sharing child care', Spare Rib, January 1980, p. 33.)

about a communal parent-run crêche set up by parents to provide each other with support and time off from child care. In the absence of good quality local authority provision, more and more of these groups are springing up. (See Chapter 7.)

ANGRY CHILDREN

When do we feel angry? When we are tired and fed up; when we feel that we have not been properly understood; when life seems to be unreasonable and unfair and, of course, when another person is deliberately rude, aggressive, or unpleasant. Children feel angry for much the same reasons. Since they have even less control over the things that happen to them than we do, they are frustrated more often and, being less inhibited or self-controlled, they let us know in no uncertain terms.

Anger is not bad behaviour – it is an expression of feeling which to that child, at that time, is perfectly valid. Some children seem to find a way of expressing their feelings very early on without indulging in fits of screaming, or they go through short periods when they are inclined to let rip at the slightest setback. Others have great difficulty in finding more socially acceptable ways of making their needs felt and lose control regularly over a long period of time.

However good the reasons for anger, we have to find ways of helping children to express their feelings, or deal with frustration, in a way which is more acceptable to everyone around them, and a lot less wearing for them – a task which would be a whole lot easier if we didn't have to deal with our own feelings at the same time.

'Usually I try distraction techniques, changing the subject, jollying along until I snap and scream at him illogically to stop screaming. Breaking point usually depends on how much sleep I got the night before.'

There can be few parents who have never responded to their child's rage by shouting back. To do so occasionally demonstrates that we, too, have strong feelings. If we do it often we may succeed in suppressing our children's angry outbursts but we will not have helped them to cope with these feelings. If a child loses control, the way to bring her back is not to lose control ourselves but to provide a space in which she can struggle to regain her dignity.

'I find now that keeping calm has a dramatic effect; whereas before I'd probably shout – now I stay calm and it's all over in a third of the time. This works if it's only me around but dealing with other adults and the tantrum is more difficult.'

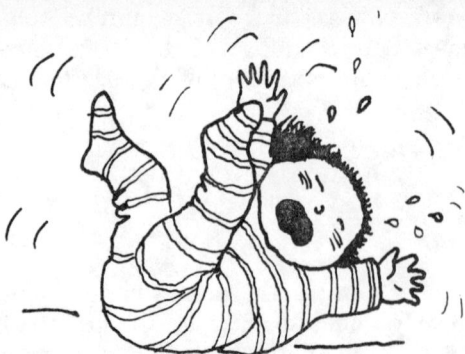

Indeed, the attitude of other adults is often more difficult to cope with than the behaviour of children:

> 'Generally the worst fits of temper are the ones that happen in public because people disapprove – of you, not the child! I remember in Cork, letting Bobby lie face down on the pavement and yell about something (which direction to go in, I think), and being glared at until I had to yank him along with me. They mainly disapproved of him getting dirty.'

Support (not interference), given at the right moment, can help when a child makes a public display of anger.

> 'We were at the toy library when a child began to have a tantrum. He was big for his age and his anger was pretty frightening. Most of the women there just drew away with their children looking terribly disapproving. His mother was in tears and clearly very upset but she was managing incredibly well. Holding him in her arms and talking quietly to him while he thrashed and kicked. In the end I went over and put my arm round her. Another couple of mothers came too and we talked to her. My oldest child had been pretty difficult too and I really felt for her.'

Looking for the cause

Furious outbursts are particularly likely between the ages of two and three when children are learning new things at a tremendous rate and loathe being frustrated. For a few this period is extended, and sometimes a child who has been even-tempered and sunny the whole way through the pre-school years starts throwing tantrums every afternoon after school. Unfair though it is, it is often a child's primary caretaker, usually his mother, who bares the brunt of this emotional teething.

*'It is not nice to be treated to a display of kicking, screaming and abuse
by someone who you love more than anything. The only consolation
is the knowledge that I am the only person in the world who he loves
and trusts enough to treat like this without fear of losing me.
Sometimes it is a pretty small consolation.'*

Just as we are more 'short-tempered' when we are feeling tired or low,
children are more likely to lose control when they are feeling particularly
hungry or tired or particularly in need of attention.

*'I would never dream of taking Matthew to a supermarket after 6 pm.
He is always tired and ratty and I know he would end up screaming.'*

Regular angry outbursts in an older child who has no particular pattern of
such behaviour, particularly if the child seems generally unhappy or hostile,
may be a signal that something is more fundamentally wrong than a passing
frustration. It may be a reaction to a period of tension between parents, a
change in caretakers, or a response to the stress of starting school or nursery.

Simply identifying the reason for a period of anger can help parents and
children come to terms with the problem (see 'Avoidable and unavoidable
stress', p.50). It may be simply that the child needs time to adjust to a new
situation and, knowing that, parents can more easily provide the support
needed to weather the storm.

*'He started having tantrums after the baby was born. That phase lasted,
on and off, for about six months. I would grab him and hold him very
closely to me and this was very effective. During these tantrums I would
be completely silent.'*

If you find it impossible to identify the cause of an extended period of
unhappiness and anger, or feel helpless about making changes, you may
want professional help. Sometimes you just need reassurance that you are
handling the situation as well as you can. (See 'How we can help each other',
p. 57–63.)

Living with tantrums

This is not a recommended strategy for coping with a tantrum but it is one
which many mothers will recognise:

*'I had never smacked Amy until she started having tantrums. It is
easier to cope with wheeling a sobbing heap round a supermarket
than a kicking, screaming monster.'*

None of us is helped by the fact that we live in a society in which children
are surrounded by things that they cannot have and places where they
cannot go. A child who has just learned that delicious things come in shiny

paper wrappers will be understandably frustrated when confronted by rows and rows of such things which she cannot touch. A child who has just learned (to great applause) that he can walk will be astonished when his parent gets upset because he wants to try out this newfound skill on a road.

But tantrums are not always about the event which appears to trigger them, and once a bout has taken hold it can rarely be stopped by giving in. Usually the need to express rage has become more important than what the rage was about. As often as not, if we give in and provide the chocolate, it will be thrown at us. Even if the rage does subside, what are we teaching our children?

'My boy used to bang his head on the floor but because I didn't give in he learned something. What do they learn from getting sweets and toys? That the more they scream the more they will get? Sweets have no educational value whatsoever and I sometimes believe that toys have no long-lasting value either. I try to give him sweets or something similar when he's good.'

It helps to be very clear and consistent about what a child can and cannot do. This at least helps her to differentiate between things and places which are off limits and those that are allowed even if, at first, she doesn't understand why.

'I have always been very clear that my children can only have sweets as occasional treats because they are bad for them. To back this up I never allow them to see me buy sweets. On the rare occasions they get them, they are "conjured out of the air". This means that, so far at least, they do not associate shopping expeditions with buying such things. It simply doesn't occur to them to ask. However I do allow them each a packet of crisps and a drink which I consider a fair recompense for being dragged around a shop full of goodies for an hour. This strategy still works with my eight year old and has worked so far with his three year old sister.'

Regular rages can sometimes be avoided with a little thought and planning. Isaac used to throw a wobbly every afternoon when his mother arrived to pick him up.

'One minute he would be a happy charming child, the next a screaming horror. The rage always centred around food. His mother had got used to breast feeding him when he cried. When she weaned him she replaced the breast with a store of food in her handbag. He expressed his demands for attention as a demand for food. The problem eased when the crèche cut off the food supply and his mother took him straight out at the end of the day instead of stopping to chat.'

Random rages are unfortunately most likely to occur when we are least able to provide calm attention. It may be that we are feeling particularly tired, or it is the week before a period and our patience is in short supply. It may be that we are hungry for company ourselves and don't recognise the warning signals.

'I think he was too tired. Being alone in London I was very aware of the terrible dependence that children had with their parents and I tried to see other women to help Paul mix with their children. This time I overdid it. I didn't know what to do. I shouted at him but in the end we just left and he screamed for a while in the street until he calmed down by himself.'

When the situation cannot be avoided you will have to find a strategy for coping.

'My toddler's worst tantrums have taken place indoors. I've learned to ignore him and sing nice songs at the top of my voice. He'd soon get up off the floor and stop crying and forget what he was wanting. If I anticipate a tantrum I usually try to distract him by getting excited about something else. I've also learned that if you talk to them and try to explain the reasons why, simply, they forget quickly about their tantrum.'

The strategy depends on the child and what is causing the anger. If a child is going off the deep end because he feels particularly needy for attention, the best strategy may be to pick him up and cuddle him. Then, when the crying stops, try to find the opportunity to give him some exclusive attention.

'One child just seemed to lose control completely. He wouldn't let you near and would just kick and struggle and shout, "I don't like you." I found it best to let him lie on a mattress and scream until he regained his self-control. Later I would find some way of letting him know that we were still friends.'

The sound of your own child screaming triggers some very powerful emotions. You want to make her better, you want the noise to stop, and you may feel rage welling up because you know that her behaviour is unreasonable and you cannot reach her. With all that going on, stepping back and dealing coolly with the situation requires some strength. We need to be able to deal with our own anger and frustration but we also have to exercise some self-control. This mother found that, by spending some time thinking about what would help her to cope with the situation, she was helping her child too.

'When she starts to scream, I go into the other room and put on some very soothing music and dance, or just lie down, depending on my mood. The sounds cut through and calm me down. At first she just raged louder and louder but because the music made me feel calmer I could cope with my own rage. Nowadays she tends to stop very soon and follow me. Often we dance together for a while and end up feeling much happier.'

Older children

As children start to be able to communicate verbally the rages often die away. If you can ask clearly for what you want then you don't have to face the irritation of coping with some stupid adult who is totally unable to understand.

However, children do not always understand exactly what it is that they want, or else they fear that their needs are totally unacceptable. It is very hard to explain to your parents that you are angry because you hate your new baby sister, or that starting nursery school has made you feel so tired that you need to go to bed an hour earlier than usual, or that a new kid in the group is being nasty to you and you cannot quite get the fear out of the back of your mind. Maybe your parents are fighting and you are afraid of the way they are behaving, or your friend's daddy has just left home and you are worried that yours will too.

Some children seem to be able to articulate their feelings very early on. They can come to terms with their fears by talking them out rather than screaming them out. Others may withdraw and turn their anger against themselves by getting depressed, sullen, hostile or difficult to communicate with. An angry child is at least getting her feelings out. The withdrawn child may need help identifying exactly what is wrong. It may help just to give a child a clear opportunity to try and figure it out by telling, or reading, stories which relate to likely areas of tension. If she can identify the problem, and know that you understand and don't condemn her, it may be a big help.

FEAR

Children can set their own limits from fear and anxiety about approaching anything new. While the parents of a 'hard-to-control' child can reassure themselves that their child is learning at breakneck speed, parents of timid children may worry that their child is simply not pushing at the boundaries or seeking independence.

Fear is basically a protective emotion. Sometimes it is instinctive: our fear of standing at the edge of a cliff is a very good way of ensuring that we don't go over the top. Sometimes it is learned: many women fear walking alone at night because they have learned, through press reports and their own experience, that women alone are vulnerable. It is sometimes based more on imagination than reality: it is unlikely that a murderous villain is hiding in that closed room. Occasionally, however, fear takes on a life of its own, controlling the way in which we live our life.

Children need to feel fear to stop them climbing too high, playing with ferocious dogs, and getting into strangers' cars. A certain amount of fear is reassuring:

*'He never showed any fear in water. When he was three he would
happily run and jump into my arms. I loved his boldness but I could
never relax for a moment in case he jumped in when I was not looking.'*

At the same time we do not want our children's fears to become barriers to
exploration, achievement and independence. Thinking a bit about our own
reaction to fear and how we cope with it may provide clues about how to
help our children cope with fear. It may also prevent us from reinforcing
fears they already have.

*'I spent years being terrified of being alone in a house at night. My fear
was perfectly logical – we had an intruder who continued to loiter at
the windows for weeks. My own experience tells me that fear cannot be
countered by logic. I would turn on the light, sit up, and work out that
the noise I could hear was my own heart beating. But I still couldn't
sleep. At that point I realised that the only way to stop the fear was to
make sure there was always someone else in the house and, if that was
not possible, to sleep elsewhere. Very, very gradually, the fear has lifted
but I know it hasn't gone altogether.'*

A child's fear of the dark feels just as 'real' as this. Just as an adult cannot
conquer fear by 'being brave', nor will a child feel less fear by being forced
to sleep with the lights off and the door shut. She will probably just become
afraid of going to bed. The bigger the fear grows the more it will occupy her
waking hours as well. It is much better to leave enough light for her to see
by if she wakes at night. You won't have tackled the reasons for her fear
but you will have stopped her from being afraid which, from her point of
view, is just as good.

Similarly, taunting a child for being a softie will not make her brave:

*'A family arrived at the pool side with a two-year-old and a baby of
about nine months. The father took the baby into the paddling pool
and she loved it. The two-year-old refused to go in the water at all.
Father started by jeering and saying "your sister doesn't mind the water
and she's only a baby." Then he forced the toddler into the big pool
where she screamed with fear and inevitably inhaled plenty of water.
The child did not go near the pool for the rest of the two weeks we were
there. She preferred to brave the contempt of her father rather than
get her feet wet.'*

Coping with fear

If a fear is clearly getting in the way of everyday life it does need to be
tackled. The child needs to be able to learn to cope with fear *himself* and to
overcome it. Many children are terrified of dogs. If this simply leads them

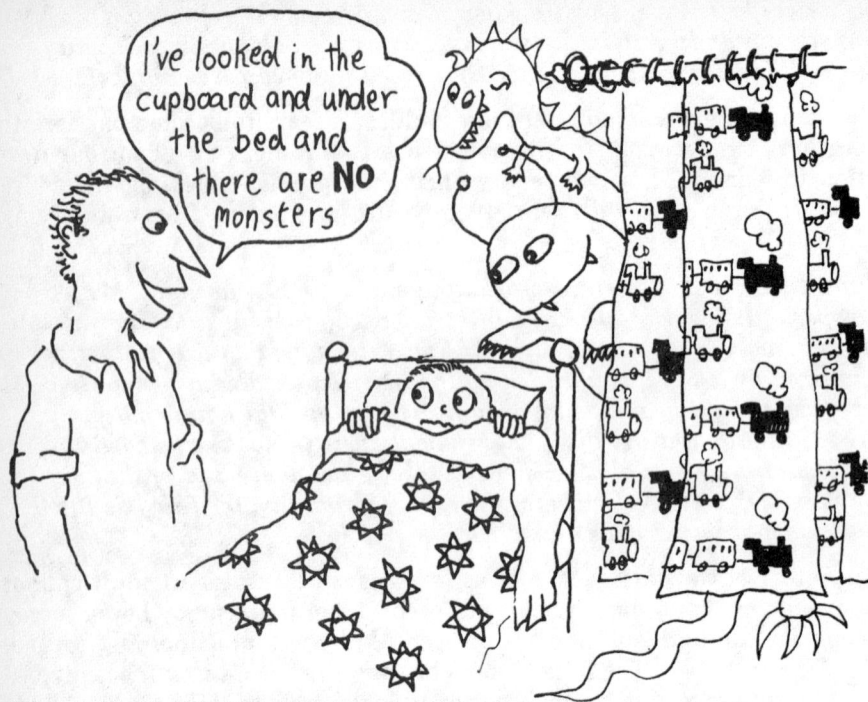

to avoid dogs no harm has been done. If the sight of a dog twenty feet away and walking in the opposite direction makes a child scream in terror, then he needs some help to deal with his fear.

'The greengrocer kept a large, but extremely gentle dog called Peaches. The children would call out for him as we passed and, though the frightened ones would stay well away, they were at least able to observe, safely, that this dog would not bite them. When we met other dogs we would make sure that we were close enough to hold on to the children who were frightened. Then they could learn that it was safe just to stand still and let the dog pass. They did not need to scream and we would keep them safe.'

Ali, an eight-year-old boy, told me how he coped with his fear of dogs:

'You just have to stand still till they pass. The main thing is not to run away. A kid on our street ran away from a dog and the dog chased it. If you stand still it won't hurt you.'

However, recognising a fear and providing reassurance is different from encouraging it. Fear is infectious. I well remember walking across a common with a friend at twilight. We were both chatting happily until, realising that it was getting dark, we looked at each other, and ran, arriving home with our hearts pounding. Had my friend been calm and unafraid I am sure I would have been able to walk the rest of the way without panicking. Realising that he was scared too doubled my fear. To our children we represent safety. If we show that we're afraid, we compound their fears.

One of the times when we are most likely to show our fear is when we leave our children with someone else for the first time. Bruno Bettelheim wisely observes that, although separation anxiety (the fear of being left by the person, or people, we depend on) is perfectly normal, we can make the problem a great deal worse if we react anxiously ourselves.

> 'Many, if not all children are a bit hesitant about the new situation of nursery school and initially have some difficulty separating from their mother. All depends on the signals the child receives; if these convey to him that this is a safe, and desirable situation, he soon contentedly enjoys the new experience. If, on the other hand, the child's initial difficulty in letting mother leave evokes responses in her which suggest to the child that she, too, is worried about what may happen, and does not wish to leave him, then initially his upset is deepened . . . it is more the mother's anxiety than the child's which keeps the process going.'

Similarly, if we react with fear every time our child climbs on a chair, and cry out with alarm the minute our toddler tumbles, we are teaching them that climbing is dangerous and falls are frightening.

> 'I have always tried to avoid reacting to my children's bumps and scrapes and falls. If they cry, I will comfort them, if the scrapes are dirty, I will clean them. If they don't seem upset I try to avoid making any comment other than a cheerful, "up you get". I know that when they do cry they really mean it and I always respond. I find that they actually cry very little, and they never put it on to get extra attention. They are also very confident about their own physical abilities. Neither of them are particularly athletic, but they have a very clear sense of what they can do and clearly see bumps and scrapes as trophies on the way to achievement rather than things to fear.'

Fear reactions can change as a child gets older. A child who is very bold at eighteen months and will climb anything that looks climbable, may be much more cautious a year later. He is learning to assess his own abilities and, for a time, may be over-cautious as he tries to work out mentally what he can achieve physically. The more opportunity he gets to practise this particular skill, with help if necessary, the sooner he will work out, for himself, just how high it is safe to go. If we provide calm reassurance we can help a child to stretch out and try something a little bit frightening. We are helping them to control fear too, and to experience the pleasure of achievement.

Chapter 4

SLEEP

Here I am in the dark alone
What is it going to be?
I can think whatever I like to think
I can play whatever I like to play.
I can laugh whatever I like to laugh.
There's nobody here but me.
(A. A. Milne, *Now We Are Six*)

SLEEP AND YOU

Sleep is the one area in which a baby's behaviour and the needs of parents come most often, and most sharply, into conflict.

'Fantasy: baby asleep in cot, mother working quietly in same room.
Reality: no sleep for four months at night, during day he napped for
no longer than twenty minutes at a time. Result: shattered, "mad"
mother unable to do the slightest chore.'

It must be wonderful to be the sort of parent who really can manage on three or four hours' sleep a night, and clean the floor and write a novel in the early hours of the morning while waiting for baby to awake. Few of us are. Most parents spend the early weeks of parenthood in a haze of tiredness. Luckily, for many of us, the haze is tinged with the pleasure of having a baby, so we stumble about feeling like death with a silly grin on our faces. But if we have insufficient support, or feel insecure about our ability to cope, tiredness can easily descend into misery and depression. If you are very tired, it is indeed hard to cope.

'I remember a feeling of total desperation. I was aching with the need
to sleep and she simply refused to settle. Soon we were both crying
with mutual frustration. Thank God I had someone to take over for a
couple of hours. That was all it took and I could cope again. That
was the worst moment.'

But it is not all bad. Our bodies and minds are extraordinarily flexible and are able to adapt to a regime which we would previously have considered impossible.

> *'Now, when I have a series of bad nights I can reassure myself. I know I will survive. I know I can get through the day and I feel a sense of pride at the fact that I have been able to adapt to such a radically different sleep pattern without literally shattering.'*

For an unlucky minority sleepless nights continue for several months or even years. Studies (e.g. Richman, 1982) show that up to 20 per cent of one- to two-year olds and 14 per cent of three-year-olds wake regularly. Given the number of people affected by sleep problems it is perhaps surprising that it is not a matter for public discussion outside the pages of baby magazines. But the general assumption is that Mummy will cope and that it doesn't matter because she can catch up with the odd nap during the day.

While it may be true that women carry most of the load of domestic nightwork, the idea that we can all catch up by napping in the day is absurd. Babies who don't sleep well at night quite often sleep badly by day as well and if the baby doesn't sleep nor can you. For those of us who have other children there is absolutely no guarantee that sleeping patterns will coincide, particularly in the early weeks, and all too often the only time you can get around to cooking or washing up is when the baby is asleep. On top of that many babies have not settled down into a night sleeping pattern before their mothers' return to work, when there is certainly no chance of a quick daily kip.

In spite of the fact that many mothers go around in the first few months feeling like a limp rag it is not uncommon for them to go to enormous lengths to protect their partners from the ill effects of sleeplessness and, as a result, absorb the entire shock of new parenthood, lapsing into a state of exhaustion and a cycle of depression which it is hard to break.

> *'The baby slept in his own room and, on waking, I had to creep into his room and sort him out so as not to wake my husband: I must have been mad.'*

If there are two of you a certain division of labour makes sense (there is not much point in both of you pacing the floor at 3 am) but there are other ways of sharing. One partner can do the night feeds and then sleep on for a couple of hours while the other gets the baby up in the morning. Similarly a partner who goes out to work can take over in the evening, and take the baby out at the weekends to make sure the main carer gets a lie-in. If you are bottle feeding you can rotate nights.

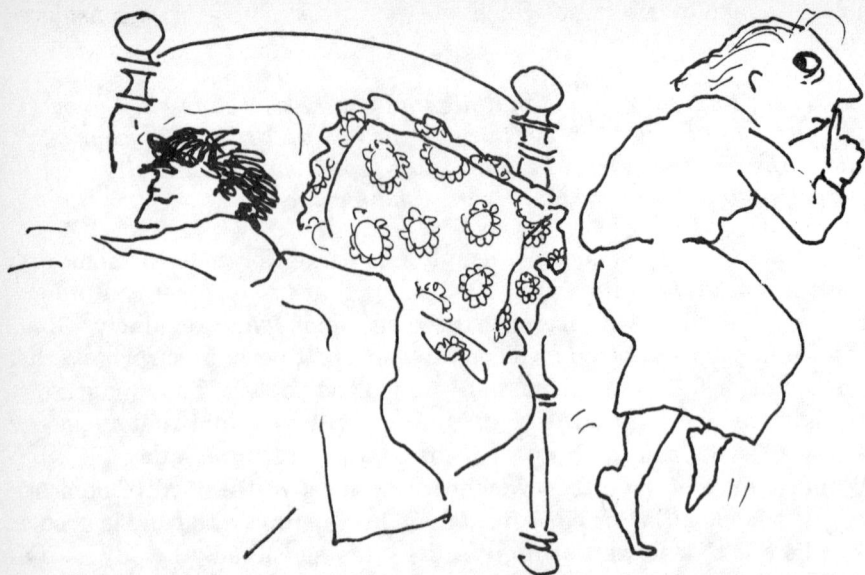

This period of real sleep disruption will probably not last more than a few weeks. If it is severe you may decide to give up most of your social pleasures for a while and concentrate your energies on surviving for as long as it takes. If after three months things have still not settled down, you may well want some help in establishing a sleep pattern you can cope with.

'I tried everything. I thought maybe he was too hot and took some covers off, then I panicked that he would be too cold and put them back on. I tried leaving a light on and turning all the lights off, I tried leaving a radio on and then I tried turning it off. In fact I tried so many things that I couldn't keep track of what I was doing. I had no idea what worked and I didn't try anything for long enough to find out.'

Sleep deprivation causes lapses in concentration and depression – a pretty fatal combination if you happen to be driving a bus, and not terribly safe if you are looking after a baby either. If anyone bothered to do research into the connection between sleep deprivation and accidents at work, the money to provide the necessary post-natal support might be forthcoming. As it is, many mothers are left to struggle on alone with conflicting advice which only seems to reinforce their sense of failure.

If you are lucky you may see a health visitor who has experience of handling sleep problems. You are more likely to get a pat on the back, perhaps a prescription for a sleeping drug, and a sense that its all your problem and your failure as a parent. What you need is encouragement in your own ability to sort things out and survive. Most of all, this means

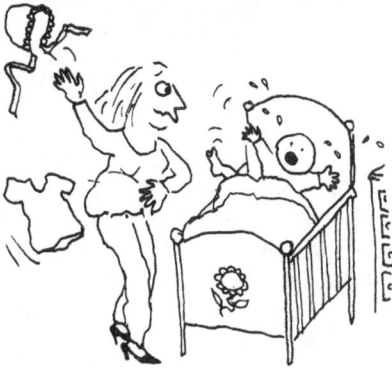

... I thought he was too hot...

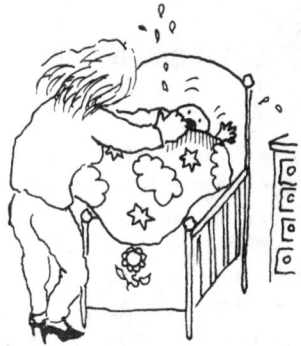

too cold...

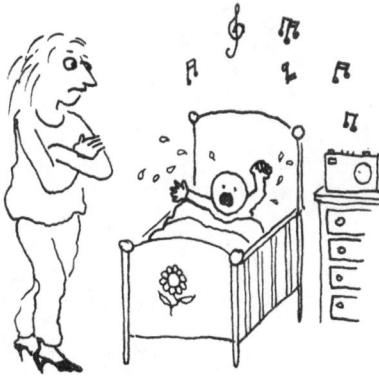

... I put on the radio...

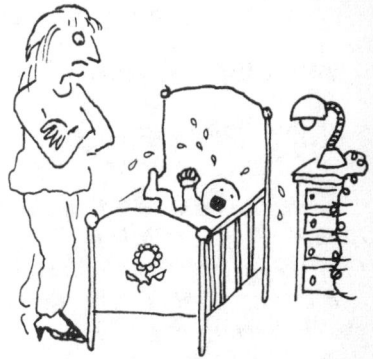

... the light...

switched it off...

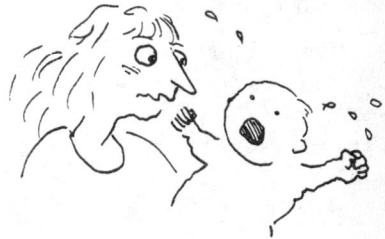

.... I couldn't keep track..

getting help in identifying just what the problem is and working out a sensible solution.

WHAT TO EXPECT AT NIGHT

A large-scale survey (Golding and Frederick, 1986) of children from birth to five discovered that by the third month most babies have settled into a pattern of being mostly asleep at night and awake by day. However, the babies did not reliably settle into a pattern of sleeping through the night until they reached eight months. Premature babies were likely to take even longer to settle down. This behaviour did not vary according to class, ethnic group, or even geography. The only factor which made any difference to whether or not children had interrupted sleep after the first few months, was the experience of their parents. Second and subsequent children tend to settle down quicker and more reliably than first ones. Nevertheless, babies do differ enormously and so do parents.

The early weeks

Some babies just seem to fall into a good pattern from Day One without any help.

'I was totally amazed that my two slept so much when they were born. Both slept in a cradle by my bedside until they were three months old then they were put into a cot in their own rooms. My eldest boy, at five and a half months went to bed at 6 pm and slept until 6 or 7 am. I put the second one to bed at 7 or 8 pm and he sleeps through until about 7 or 8 the following morning.'

Others need a lot of reinforcement before they adapt to a sleeping pattern which faintly resembles your own.

'Matthew was born in the early evening. That meant he had his most wakeful newborn phase just as I was trying to go to sleep. In fact he slept very little that first night. During the next day he got his recovery sleep – I did not. For the next few days the pattern was the same. He simply did not want to sleep at night. By the eighth day I was really wondering whether I was losing my mind.'

Babies may have attacks of indigestion, particularly in the evening, and may be very unsettled. A doctor reported:

'Our third baby was the most difficult. He screamed for the longest between 11 pm and 3 am. Experience helped in that I understood that

there was nothing wrong with him, it was just the way he was, but it was still hard to deal with – you expect to be able to get your baby to sleep.'

What one set of parents may consider absolute torture, their neighbours will cope with quite happily for years.

'None of my four children had a whole night's sleep during their first two years. I got used to this routine and never had the tired syndrome.'

If your baby is very unsettled you might try using a pram as a bed at night so that you can provide the motion that may lull her to sleep. Some babies feel much happier when they can hear a constant background noise. Tapes are available of the sounds that babies hear in the womb, and these can be very effective, but just leaving a radio on low may be enough. These techniques are all short-term measures but they can provide invaluable support for a baby who is learning to sleep alone. (For more about crying babies see p. 84.)

From cradle to cot

Parents tend to transfer babies from their bed, or from a cradle to a cot, at about three months and, if they have the space, into a separate room when they start to sleep reliably. One mother set herself a clear guideline:

'Both babies began by sleeping in a cot by my bedside. When the night feeds dropped to no later than midnight and no earlier than 5 am I moved them to their own room.'

If your baby is already sleeping soundly and is used to going to sleep on her own, the transition will probably not be difficult. A baby who has been used to snuggling up against a warm parent at night may not take kindly to being transferred and may demand to be taken back in during the night. If you want to put a stop to this, there are ways of doing so which are discussed below.

From cot to bed

This may be a step you want to postpone if you think your child will take to wandering at night. It is probably worthwhile trying to tackle problems of night waking or difficulty settling at bedtime (see below) while your child is still cot-bound. However, some children force the issue by learning to climb out of their cots at around two years old. Since this can be a rather dangerous activity it may be better to abandon the cot altogether or, at least, lower the side. Others cling to their cots and seem reluctant to make the transition.

> 'When I suggested that Ruth transfer to the bottom bunk she was surprisingly reluctant. I left the cot up next to the bunk for a few days, and then suggested that we try again. When I put the ladder next to her to stop her falling out the space seemed more contained and she crawled in quite happily. I never had the problem I feared that she would simply get out of bed and refuse to go to sleep.'

Thinking about your needs

Most books start with the needs of the baby and then expect you to adapt. The only problem with this approach is that it doesn't take into consideration the interaction between parents and children. If you can cope with being roused from a deep sleep several times a night and still be calm and loving during the day, then you can afford to let the baby's needs and preferences set the agenda.

> 'If any of them cried I could, and would, go to him and hold him. I never minded bringing them into bed with me.'

If sleep deprivation makes you foul-tempered and weepy both you and your child will probably benefit from a more managed approach. Establishing a system which allows you to get a few hours of uninterrupted oblivion at night is not, as many baby books suggest, an infringement of your baby's individual rights but a matter of your own sane survival. You need to sleep so therefore you must work out a way of making it possible. Your way may not be anything like your neighbours' and may be quite different from your mother's. Sleep solutions are not a matter of morality. The best way is the way that works.

In bed

In the early weeks your major concern may well be to avoid having to get up many times in the night to feed your baby. Many people manage this stage by having the baby in bed with them:

> 'During the breastfeeding period they slept with me. I couldn't and didn't want to cope with getting up and going to the child two or three times every night: none of them was ever squashed!'

Indeed, this approach to early breastfeeding is now endorsed by the Royal College of Midwives, whose current policy encourages hospitals to allow 'bedding in' as they call it – something which not too long ago was officially frowned upon as a possible source of cross-infection. However, not everyone feels comfortable with a baby in the bed.

'For nearly four years he would end up in our bed nearly every night. This would make us irritable as he would kick us all night long. I did things differently with the next two children and now I feel that you should never let children into your bed. It starts a bad habit.'

By the bed
An alternative for parents who find it hard to sleep with the baby is to have a basket or cot close to the bed, so that you can feed easily at night without getting out of bed. Parents often end up with a mixture of the two.

'I found interruption very easy to cope with as long as the baby fell asleep again quickly (usually I fell asleep again first with the baby on the breast).'

Out of the room
Very light sleepers may find that they do better with the baby in a different room, even though it means getting up to feed.

'We had our first baby in the room with us for a month. I was jumping in and out of bed half the night until we went to stay with friends whose baby slept in a separate room. I was very anxious about leaving him so far away (virtually next door!) but was converted pretty quickly when, for the first time, he slept all night. I think I had been woken by his every snuffle and I was disturbing him. When I couldn't hear him snuffle he just went back to sleep again. I had our second baby in the room next door from the fourth day and she slept pretty well.'

Compromising
If your child continues to wake at night beyond the newborn stage you may have to consider again your feelings about sharing your bed. Many parents find that once they have accustomed their child to going to bed alone, so that they have the privacy of their own bed in the first part of the night, they don't really mind if a sleepy body wriggles in between them in the early hours.

'She has a low bed to make it easy for her to get in and out but she complains that it's cold. She often sleeps in our bed, which we don't mind, except that she fidgets.'

However, you may feel very anxious and invaded by the idea of sharing your bed in this way. It can be a real bone of contention between partners, because of its implications for your privacy and in particular your sexual relationship. On the other hand it may simply be impossible to sleep if your baby wriggles and kicks. One compromise may be to keep your own bed private but sleep with your child.

*'Neither of us could cope with his night waking. Nor could we sleep
with him in the bed. One of us would stumble in, try to get him back
to sleep and more often than not, crash out next to him. He would sleep,
we would sleep. It wasn't until he was nearly three that we made any
serious attempt to stop his waking.'*

If you definitely do not want to indulge in night-time musical beds but your
child feels differently, there are ways of managing these difficulties discussed
below.

Setting a bedtime

You may not be at all concerned with getting your children to bed at a set
time. Indeed, if you work all day you may positively prefer keeping them up
with you late in the evening:

*'She goes to bed not much before we do. I think we have encouraged
her to stay up as we would otherwise never see her. As it is we get
several hours' play every evening.'*

However, if you cherish a few hours of peace and privacy in the evening,
you will want a reasonably regular bedtime. Don't expect it to happen
straight away. In the first couple of months babies are very often more alert
in the evenings than at other times of day. You may need to work at
gradually setting bedtime a little earlier over a period of time. Most people
I talked to agreed on one point:

*'Going to bed rituals are important. They don't have to be lengthy but
need to be consistent, e.g. into bed, arrange teddies, a little talk, read
a story, kisses and maybe a goodnight song. And no getting up after
that unless it's a sensible reason.'*

The young baby
It's never too early to start this pattern by, for example, always bathing
your baby last thing in the evening, changing him or her into night clothes,
giving the last feed with the lights low, or off, and leaving the baby in a
quiet room. It is tempting to allow a baby to drop off while feeding and then
quietly transfer her to bed. However, studies of children with sleep problems
show the value of allowing babies to drop off to sleep in the place where
they are going to spend the night, rather than in your arms. This way, if
they stir later on, they will know where they are and not wake up in a
fright.

Even if your baby shares your bed it may help to ensure that she learns
to go to sleep without your assistance. If she always falls asleep on your
breast she may keep stirring and, finding that the nipple has disappeared,

cry out until you wake and give it back to her. As a tiny baby she assumes that your breast is part of her so it must be pretty disconcerting to fall asleep firmly attached to this rather nice bit of body and wake up to find it missing. Dummies may present a similar problem. If it falls out the baby cannot put it back in and cries for help.

Establishing a routine doesn't mean you have to stick to it slavishly. You will usually find that the occasional evening out at a friend's house can be managed without problems. You have to make your own decision how much disruption you and your child can cope with.

'We got Sue to go to bed on her own almost from the start and she would quite happily sleep in her own room. We could also take her out in the carrycot at night now and then without upsetting her routine. What we couldn't do was allow her downstairs after bed time without "paying" for it. If she cried in the evening and we gave in and brought her downstairs she would "create" for a week, until we convinced her that we were not going to do it again.'

Some people decide to let the babies routine dictate their own organisation:

'I think that a regular routine can be limiting for the carer but I have decided its the price I'm prepared to pay for the time to myself that it gives me. She goes to bed at 6.30 and sleeps through until around 8 am. She has never been particularly portable but I don't like to take her in the evenings anyway.'

Single parents may have particular difficulties in establishing a routine because it is hard to go out unless you take the baby too and staying in can be very lonely. Once again you will need to work out the balance which suits you. If your baby cries all evening and won't settle when you go out it may be in your interests to stay in for a while until you work out a way to get your baby to settle more easily. Nothing is for ever with a baby. The chances are, when you have a pattern worked out, and you and your baby are more relaxed, going out will be easy again.

Older babies and children
Even good sleepers may start kicking up a fuss about going to bed when they are slightly older. When a baby learns for the first time to stand it can trigger a problem settling at nights:

'Ruth learned to stand while we were on holiday. She was so pleased with herself that, when I put her to bed, she would just get up again and yell. If she woke at night we would have the same routine.'

If you just continue as usual, putting your baby to bed and leaving the room as you have always done, you can then return every now and again with a few calm, reassuring words, lie her down and cover her up, until eventually

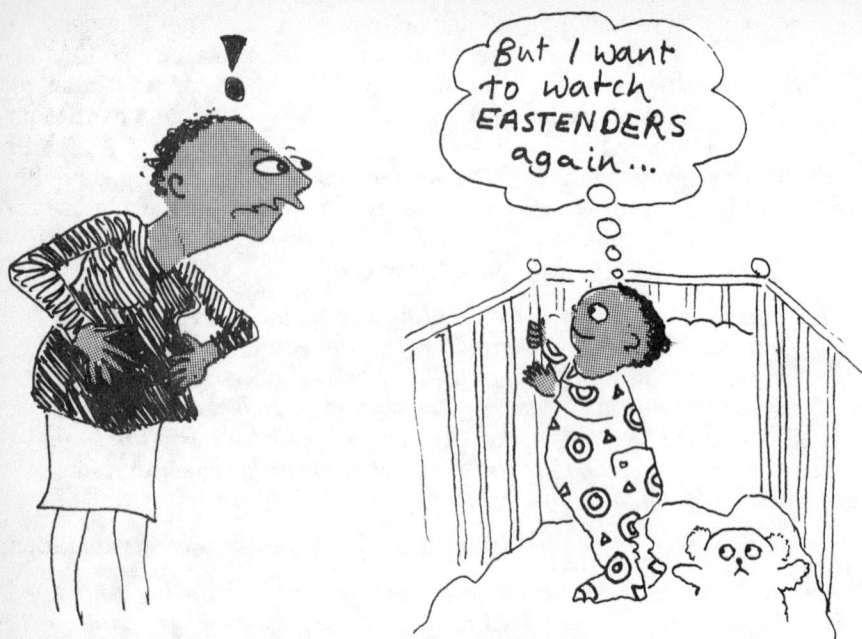

she is tired and gives up. Over a few days the old pattern will probably be re-established. With a cot-bound baby it is fairly easy to take effective action. You know your baby is able to sleep alone and knows what it is all about. It is just a question of waiting it out until this new phase dies away.

The same problem may occur when you first move your baby from a cot to a bed.

> 'He just would not let me leave the room. I would sit by him and he would fasten his arms firmly around my neck. If I tried to move he would stir and tighten his grip. I had to sit there until he was totally asleep and then gradually loosen his grip and wriggle out.'

Once your child is in a bed it is obviously not so easy but, once again, a calm and consistent approach will usually work.

Re-establishing a routine can take a few days, which will infuriate you if it starts on the day you had planned to go to a movie or just before your favourite TV programme. If you break your own rules and bring your child downstairs to sit on your knee while you watch the programme you would otherwise miss, he will expect the same reward for his behaviour tomorrow. If you have a partner you can take turns at putting the child to bed. If not, you could try setting bedtime half an hour earlier to give yourself a longer wind-down and more time to settle him. Children have an uncanny way of knowing when you desperately want them to settle because you are going out or have some other appointment. On those days give yourself plenty of time.

Fear of the dark

Some children suddenly start to be afraid of going to bed for no apparent reason. The most likely age for this is between four and five. They may be afraid of the dark or perhaps they have frightened themselves with stories about monsters. A night light may be very reassuring for a genuinely frightened child and a ritual that includes checking under the bed and in the cupboards for monsters may reassure him that all is well. Talking about fears usually helps to put them into proportion (see 'Fear', pp. 68–71) but the aim, in the end, must still be to help the child to fall asleep happily in his own bed.

WHAT TO EXPECT BY DAY

It is a rare baby who does not need to sleep during the day in the first year. On the other hand, there are many babies who apparently prefer to catnap.

'Inevitably he would sleep during shopping, or in the park (when mother was staggering around in a twilight world), but not when I could rest.'

'He didn't sleep in the day until he could crawl, then he settled into a two sleep a day routine.'

A baby who refuses to go to sleep during the day may well be a baby who is also quite hard to settle to sleep in the evening, and the problem may well be the same: the baby is too tired and wound-up to settle. Tired babies and toddlers, like tired adults, may be pretty bad company. Organising a sleep routine for the day will give you some time to yourself and make your hours together more rewarding. It helps to put a child to bed as soon as she seems a little sleepy rather than waiting for her to get wound up from exhaustion.

'What I didn't realise was how much sleep she needed in the day too. She would cry for hours in the afternoon and I would try to jolly her along, not realising that she was crazy for another sleep. A good friend had told me that this might happen but it still took weeks until I realised what was happening. Now (at eighteen months) she has two naps of 1½ hours in the day and sleeps for around 13½ hours at night. We now keep to a strict routine.'

As a general rule it is best to allow a baby or toddler to keep a regular daytime sleep until she simply stops sleeping when you put her to bed, which usually happens anywhere between two years and starting school. However, this can be a problem if a long midday sleep means that she is too full of energy to go to sleep at night. If you decide to stop your child sleeping in the day in order to improve things at night, the period of weaning off the midday sleep can be pretty grim. Your child may be thoroughly bad-tempered all afternoon and, if she is too over-tired, she may well sleep badly at night too. You could try allowing a short afternoon sleep and then waking her. Some toddlers wake in an absolutely vile mood if you do this, but persist for a while – they often get used to it. Alternatively allowing a sleep on alternate days may be a better compromise.

COPING WITH SLEEP PROBLEMS

Crying babies

If your baby is miserable and unsettled in the evening all the above must sound like pie in the sky. It may be hard to imagine that you will ever be able to put your baby to bed and calmly leave the room. Some babies cry all evening because they are tired. If this is the case you may well find that the baby you have been jiggling and rocking for a couple of hours just wants to be left in peace. After a few minutes of protest she may drop off gratefully:

'It was his dad who tried it first. I was trying to make a meal which was impossible because the baby kept crying. I would pick him up and feed him and then put him down and he would just wake up again. He took him away and put him to bed in another room with the light off and two doors shut between him and me. I was certain I could still hear him crying and after five minutes insisted that we go and check. He was fast asleep. After that I put him down and let him cry himself to sleep every night. It never took more than a few minutes and then he would sleep for twelve hours straight.'

It may also be that your milk supply (if you are breast feeding) is at a low ebb in the evening after a busy day. Look at 'A lactation diet' (p. 96) for more on increasing your milk supply.

Cutting daytime sleep may not help at all. If your baby is overtired she may work herself up into a frenzy which will make it even harder to settle her.

Some babies really do cry out of discomfort, often for hours at a time, and nothing seems to help. In some cases the problem can be traced to an allergy (see 'Allergy and food intolerance,' pp. 121–7), or it may even be a urinary infection or an ear infection, so it is worth asking your doctor to check. If you fail to discover a cause, you will probably just have to find a way of bolstering your confidence as parents until your baby grows out of this difficult phase, which she undoubtedly will. What you need most is to try and keep calm – not an easy task. Most babies are calmed by motion. A baby sling, which allows you to keep your baby strapped to your back as you move may give you some respite.

It may help you to cope with these evenings if you can manage to carve out some time in the day when you know you can be alone and relaxed. If you have a partner it will probably help both of you if you can give each other time off: perhaps for a quiet drink at a pub with a friend or even a long relaxing bath. If you are alone maybe a friend could help out by taking the baby for a walk in the pram while you get a complete break – even for half an hour.

If you have no support at all, speak to your health visitor. Although they do not have many resources these are the sorts of circumstances when they have a clear responsibility to try and provide help. One mother I know who spent every day at home, usually unaided, with triplets, got invaluable help from a health visitor who would babysit once a week so that she could get out.

Even during the unsettled times it is worth trying to establish some kind of bedtime routine. If your baby screams every night between 11 pm and 3 am you will just want to flop into bed when she drops off. As soon as you start to see a recognisable pattern emerge it is probably worthwhile trying to set up some kind of routine, however brief. That way your baby knows that you will stay with her when she needs you but that bedtime is still bedtime.

Cry-sis provides a help line for desperate parents. If you are finding it hard to cope with a crying baby, don't blame yourself, don't assume you have done something wrong and don't be afraid to ask for help. Also read Sheila Kitzinger's *The Crying Baby* (Viking, 1989).

Children who wake

We all expect our newborn babies to wake during the night for feeds. If after five months or more, on three solid meals a day, your baby is still waking regularly two or three times a night, you may start feeling rather fed up.

'Will was still waking every three hours at the age of two. What's more he would only go back to sleep if I breastfed him. I was like a zombie.'

You may discover, ironically, that it is the feeds which are causing the waking. It doesn't matter whether it's breast or bottle, the effect is much the same: the baby is used to a nice uninterrupted sleepy snuggle several times a night so he or she wakes up regularly to get it. If you stop providing the reward, you may well find that, after initial protest, the waking stops. It may help if the non-feeding partner takes over at this time.

'After thirteen months, when he had finished wanting breast in the early hours, sleep went quite well – thanks to my friend Anna who told my husband that he had got to go into him with a drink of water instead of me.'

It may sound simple but of course it is not, particularly if you have no partner to turn to for support. When her twins reached five months and still weren't sleeping through the night Julia decided that she would just have to crack the sleeping problem in order to survive:

'My mum came to stay with me for a few days and that gave me the moral support I needed. Then I just put them to bed at 7 pm and left them crying for ten minutes. I used to sit outside their room with a watch and wait. If after ten minutes they seemed to be getting quieter then I would leave them a little longer. I did the same thing if they woke during the night. It was agony but within a week it worked. They slept and didn't disturb me and we were all much happier in the day.'

Worse still, your baby may have been sleeping angelically all night and then suddenly start waking every hour or so. When you have got used to sleeping properly the interruptions may be particularly upsetting. Freda's father took some pride in the fact that he had established a clear routine for his daughter. Then, at twenty months, she took to waking all through the night and wanting to get into bed with her parents. Sarah who lived with them, described the scene:

'We sat around reading every book we could find, trying to work out what to do. Then it occurred to us that she might be worrying about losing her mother. She had just applied for a new job and friends kept dropping in and saying "Are you going to Bradford?" As far as Freda was concerned, Bradford was the place her mother went without her. You forget that at that age she can understand a great deal more than she can say.'

Having found a possible cause they all felt more able to relax and just weather it until Freda felt reassured that her mother was not going to leave. Sure enough, within a week, the crisis was over. With Matthew the problem was simple to pinpoint but not so easy to cure.

'When we split up his father had the children every other weekend and one night during the week. Matthew was two years old. He didn't understand what was happening and was very unhappy. When he stayed with his father he would sleep at night. When he came home

*he was distraught and would wake up all through the night just to
make sure that I was there. It took several months for him to get used
to the new arrangement and settle at night. I was absolutely exhausted.'*

It may not be as easy as this to pinpoint the reason for a child's waking.
Before three months it is almost always attributed to wind pains. If it starts
between three and four months parents often see it as a signal to start on
solids, assuming that the problem is hunger. This may help if indeed hunger
was the cause. By four to five months, teething is usually the stock assumption. Some babies do get slightly feverish, with rather red cheeks and often
loose stools too, when they are teething. If you think your baby is feverish
and genuinely suffering discomfort, half a teaspoon of paracetamol mixture
will help. However, don't make it a habit as this mother did, quoted in *From
Here to Maternity* (Pelican, 1981) by Ann Oakley:

*'He was going through a bad patch. I think it was his teeth. We gave
him some medicine. My sister said it knocked them out. About a
month he's been having it. Every day, four times a day, in his milk.'*

This mother ended up putting paracetamol liquid (heavily sugared) in a
dinky feeder every time her baby cried – a modern-day version of the opiate
drugs which mothers gave to their babies a hundred years ago. Then, as
well as today, there may be nothing specific wrong:

*'I tried everything from a bottle to juice, teething gel, gripe water – you
name it, I did it. I don't think feeding routines make any difference. If
they are going to have sleepless nights, they will. With my daughter I
didn't know anything and sometimes felt like I couldn't cope. As soon
as she cried I was there so she expected me to be there. I let Mitchell
cry and most times he went back to sleep.'*

No matter what the cause of regular waking the solutions will be the same.
Either keep the child with you at night to give total, all-round, wall to wall
reassurance (you can perhaps postpone the issue of getting the child back
into her own bed until the particular crisis has passed), or be very calm and
very consistent and keep putting the child back down. It is best, as far as
possible, to avoid anything such as a bottle, drink (other than water), or
even a cuddle, which might be seen as a reward for waking. Your quiet voice
and perhaps a reassuring stroke should be enough to remind her that you
are there.

WHEN NOTHING SEEMS TO WORK

Maybe you have tried everything mentioned above and still nothing works.
Don't panic. Sleep problems can be solved. The first step is to decide how

bad the problem is and what kind of action you are prepared to take to change things. If there are two of you you will need to agree on this, because you will need each others support to carry it out. It may be that the problem is not actually loss of sleep but your sense of failure about not 'getting it right'. Or it may be that partners disagree about how to cope and that the tension between the two of you is the bigger problem.

'I was determined not to allow our second child to get into the habit of coming into our bed. Her father didn't care. He slept fine with her in the bed. I didn't sleep at all. Finally after a screaming row at about 3 am we decided to talk to a child psychologist specialising in sleep problems. She very quickly helped me to realise that the major problem was not our daughter's behaviour but my anxiety about it. Once I stopped minding, I relaxed, and we could all sleep.'

There are techniques for modifying children's behaviour but they are easier to manage when the child is old enough to cooperate and to get a sense of achievement out of it. Just knowing that there will come a time when your child will leave your bed might give you enough reassurance to cope with the current difficulties. However, if you are all running ragged, you may prefer the short-term disruption of making a real effort to change things, to the long-term prospect of disturbed sleep. If you are both clear about the need to modify your child's behaviour, rather than your own sleeping arrangements, there are some fairly clear steps you can take.

1) Write a sleep diary for a week. Enter every time your child sleeps, for how long, what sort of mood she is in on waking, who goes to her and exactly how you respond. This will give you a clear baseline against which you can monitor future behaviour.

2) Prepare a sleep chart, with a box for every day, so that you can monitor visually the pattern of your child's sleep when you start the sleep programme. If your child is old enough to understand what you are doing, put the chart on his bedroom wall.

Babies and toddlers
For a pre-verbal, or barely verbal, child the techniques used are based on a gradual withdrawal of parental attention at night. The speed of withdrawal depends on what you feel that you can cope with. Whatever you do, you should expect things to get much worse initially, so it may be best to wait for a time when neither of you are too heavily committed at work and will be able to cope with feeling like death.

It would not be sensible to start the programme until you are sure that your baby no longer needs night feeds from a nutritional point of view. If he is healthy and growing well, and is eating solid foods by day, night feeds should not be necessary. What is lost at night can be made up during the day.

The assumption behind a sleep programme is that you are inadvertently rewarding your child for night waking and that you have to change the way you respond so that you are no longer encouraging this behaviour. So you must look very carefully at the things you do to help your child settle back to sleep. Very often children will only settle if one particular caretaker goes to them and often settling includes a feed or a cuddle or quite lengthy rocking. This means that one parent, very often the mother, is forced to take on the whole routine of settling at bedtime and during the night.

To break the pattern it will help if the other partner (assuming there is one) takes over. The way you settle your baby at bedtime may be the crucial link. If you get that right, the later nighttime interruptions may disappear. If you are on your own, or have little support from your partner, it may be a lot less stressful if you start your new settling routine with daytime naps. Whenever you decide to start, give yourself time. You will not have the patience to go through with the programme if you are trying to get off to a meeting, or have friends to dinner. And once you do start it really is important to carry the programme through. If you slip back you will end up feeling demoralised and your child's erratic sleep pattern may have been reinforced.

Start by setting a clear bedtime routine that you know you can stick to. Tell your child what you are doing even if you don't think he can understand you. The firmness of your voice will indicate that something has changed. Then put your child to bed, tuck him in, and leave the room. You can go back every few minutes to reassure him that you are still around, speak firmly but not angrily and leave again, but do not pick him up. Some people maintain that going back simply makes things worse and that it is easier just to leave the child to cry himself to sleep. It is for you to decide what you can manage.

If the child can get out of bed and follow you, you may have to modify this technique by staying in the room but simply ignoring him once you have said goodnight. It might help to have a chair and a night light so that you can read while he drops off. Whatever you do, it must be made clear by your behaviour that you are not going to let the child get up, and you are not going to cuddle, rock or feed him to sleep.

Some people find that once the child has got the message about going to bed alone, the night waking stops too. If it doesn't you will have to deal with that separately, You can wait until you have solved the early settling problem before tackling the waking or you can do both together.

If you give your child a bottle or breast feed at night you will have to brace yourself for what could be a few hard nights. The reason you are giving these treats is to settle the child quickly to sleep, so you know that removing them will be hard. Nevertheless you will have to be firm with yourself and your child. You could try switching to a bottle of water, or very dilute juice, as a first step and then gradually reduce the volume. If this doesn't work you may simply have to cut the bottle out.

If your treat has been to take him into your bed, you could try giving him a teddy or soft cloth to cuddle. It probably won't help much but it may make you feel better. Then, when he wakes, just come in, put him down, cover him up and leave the room. He will almost certainly cry and be distressed. Leave him for as long as you can manage (five to ten minutes for example) and then go back, repeat the action and leave again. It can take several hours to settle a child this way, but if you are consistent, within a few nights your child will stop waking up.

Pre-school children

The best way to change a small child's behaviour is by gaining his cooperation. You may have to use some of the techniques described earlier, but with older children you can give clear, positive, reinforcement for desirable behaviour. The sleep chart mentioned earlier should be put on the child's wall with big squares for every day. You can then promise the child a brightly coloured sticker on the chart for every night she stays in her own bed. If it is early mornings you are trying to deal with, the sticker chart can be used alongside a large clock. Mark the time when your child can come into your room and explain that, when the hands arrive at the marks, it is morning and she can have a sticker. Talk about the chart and explain its purpose clearly. It is important never to use it for any other purpose or to deny stickers for any other reason.

You may well find that your child's behaviour changes quite dramatically and then slips back again, or that there are no stickers on the chart for a while as the child protests against the new regime. You will find that it helps you too to have the chart displayed on the wall. You can keep referring to it at bedtime, allow your child to choose the sticker she will get if she manages to stay in bed and, if progress seems slow, you can reassure yourself by comparing the chart with your pre-treatment diary. If you are having no progress at all perhaps you should make an easier first step. Read the section above, and withdraw a little more gradually. There are books specifically dealing with sleep problems listed at the back of the book on p. 215.

NIGHTMARES, NIGHT TERRORS AND SLEEPWALKING

Nightmares

These are very common, particularly for three- and four-year-olds. They occur in the lightest phase of sleep so that they usually wake the child up and seem very vivid and real. It is likely that even very young children have nightmares, but, as they cannot explain, we do not know. Usually a child will only need reassuring and comforting in order to go quite happily back to sleep.

A mind that is very active during the day may pick up a jumble of impressions that are quite disturbing at night. Monsters and wild animals make wonderful ideas for daytime play but take bigger and more colourful shape in dreams. Children who are overtired or anxious are also more likely to be woken by dreams. It may help to avoid activities which stimulate scary thoughts just before bedtime and organise a quiet wind-down time.

A child who has been through a particularly disturbing event may well have 'bad dreams' for some time until the fear or anxiety is resolved. You can only give reassurance. A night light may help or your child may ask to sleep in your bed. You will need to judge for yourself whether you feel that this would help her to cope more quickly with whatever is bothering her, realising that if she starts to sleep with you, she may be reluctant to return to her own bed.

Night frights and sleepwalking

These occur when a child is very deeply asleep. The child is unlikely to wake up and the next morning will have no recollection of what happened. In fact this behaviour is generally a lot more alarming to parents than to the children themselves.

'It's the most terrifying experience. She would be totally disorientated. She seemed to be awake and would be talking wildly but there would be no way of penetrating her consciousness. Then she would suddenly yawn and be totally calm and sleep for the rest of the night. There was a time when it happened a couple of times a week. Now, at eight years old, it is more like once a month. It never seemed to be related to any outward problems. When we were going through the most difficult times there was no increase in the frequency of these terrors.'

Since you cannot make contact with a child who is deeply asleep there is very little you can do except to reassure yourself and try to stay calm. It is not advisable to wake the child up. The fright will pass of its own accord and you can then tuck her in, or carry her back to bed. If the child is moving about you will have to take precautions to ensure that she does not damage herself. Make sure the house is safe. Children who sleepwalk are capable of negotiating stairs and doors so it is wise to lock your front door and windows, and perhaps put bolts on the outside of doors to other rooms and put up a stair-gate to restrict her access. In time your child will grow out of this phase.

Chapter 5

WHAT GOES IN

What is the matter with Mary Jane?
She's crying with all her might and main,
And she won't eat her dinner – rice pudding again –
What *is* the matter with Mary Jane?
(A. A. Milne, *When We Were Very Young*)

IN THE BEGINNING: THE FOOD OF LOVE

'I expected to hate it but those dark midnight hours were some of the most wonderful I have experienced. The warm physical presence of a baby in my arms, the smell of her skin and her hair, the rhythmic sucking and the utter peace and silence. It was worth waking up for.'

Feeding a new baby is not just about food – it is about love, anxiety, sleep and sleeplessness. Feeding will never be easier, or harder, again. When we put a baby to our breast we are not just giving milk – we are giving ourselves. It is an extraordinarily intimate relationship and, like most intimate relationships, it can be wonderful or it can fail to take off at all.

Those of us who start out intending to breastfeed and find it impossible will almost certainly feel a sense of loss for an experience missed, but there are gains too:

'Josh slept better than any breastfed babies born at the same time. We bonded away perfectly cheerfully, gazing as passionately at each other as if we were doing the REAL THING. And of course I could let someone else feed him too. Gavin also engaged in passionate gazing (could this be why he and Josh are so mutually devoted now? Did they bond better than most babies and dads?), and we could both go out together leaving the bottle behind very easily. In fact if it wasn't for worries about the baby's health I would heartily recommend it.'

So are we damaging children irretrievably if we bottle-feed? I talked to one mother who had breastfed three babies through all sorts of stress and strains and then found herself unable to feed the fourth. As she observes:

*'It's the baby that's important at the end of the day. Breastfeeding is
not best for your baby if it is not working and the baby is not putting
on weight.'*

Infant formulas are probably the most carefully manufactured foods that
exist. They are made to be as close to mothers' milk as the imperfections of
manufacturing can possibly get. As the mother above points out:

*'Ironically my bottle-fed baby has turned out to be the best eater and
the most robust of the four of them.'*

Nevertheless, she would also agree that breast milk is best for babies and,
if it's working well, has plenty to recommend it to mothers too.

WHY BREASTFEED?

From the day your baby is born until the day he or she leaves home there
is only one basic piece of advice about food: stick with products which are
as fresh as you can manage and have as little as possible added and as little
as possible taken away. Fresh, whole foods, untampered with by the wonders
of high technology, are made up of a complex mixture of different nutritional
components. We do not know exactly what they all are and we do not know
exactly what they all do. Until we know that, the safest bet is to eat foods
as close as possible to the way they grew. That way you will get everything
that they are meant to contain and a lot less of what they should not.

* Breast milk contains proteins and carbohydrates in exactly the right
  balance for a human baby. Cow's milk contains more protein per ounce
  (after all, baby cows are a lot bigger than baby humans). Cow's milk
  must therefore be changed significantly before it is suitable for a human
  baby. Milk made from soya beans is even further from being a 'whole'
  product, and is heavily sugared to make it closer in energy composition
  to human milk. It also contains a high level of aluminium which, in
  large concentrations, is poisonous.
* Some children are allergic to the protein in cow's milk (and some are
  allergic to soya protein too). There is some evidence that, in families
  with a history of allergy (eczema and asthma), avoiding cow's milk for
  the first four to six months could provide protection. (This is discussed
  more under 'Allergies', pp. 121–7).
* Antibodies built up in a mother's blood to protect against disease will
  be passed on through breast milk and provide some protection during
  the early months when babies are at their most vulnerable.
* Breast milk is more hygienic. Mixing and preparing bottle feeds is
  always a hazardous procedure. You must ensure that the water is boiled
  and that the containers are scrupulously clean and sterile or you risk

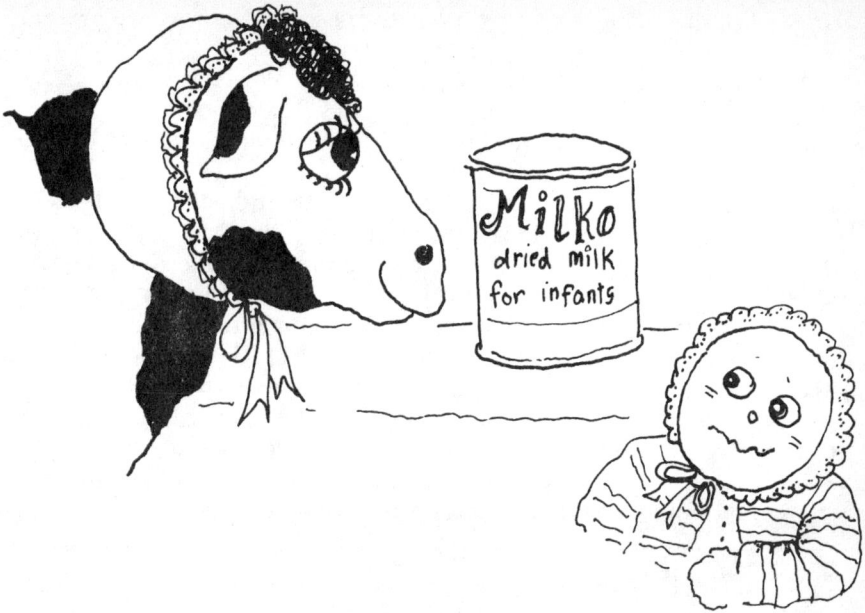

triggering a stomach upset. Breastfed babies rarely suffer from severe gastric infections.

* Breast milk is the original convenience food: no messing around with mixing, cooling and warming up again.

WHAT KEEPS US FROM BREASTFEEDING?

Public attitudes

' *"You can't do that here," Anna Bowman was told by the restaurant superviser at Harrods' cafeteria. Anna was breastfeeding her five-month-old baby. A few weeks later fifteen women sat down to tea in the same restaurant and proceeded to suckle their babies. The staff watched disapprovingly but did not interfere.*'

This press report appeared in the magazine *Spare Rib* in 1980. Nine years later the cafeteria's policy had changed little. Basically they feel that the practice is 'embarrassing and offensive to many'. These days mothers would be directed to the baby feeding and changing facilities on another floor. Bared breasts are fine, it seems, if they are on hoardings and inside newspapers, but when they are being used to provide food for a baby they must be hidden away. Female bodies can only be used for the purpose of sexual titillation.

To suggest that there might be any other purpose for the way we are made is considered embarrassing.

It isn't surprising then that many women in Western countries have taken to bottle-feeding. If to breastfeed means to lock yourself away in private communion with your child then the liberated option must be to use a bottle so that you can at least be part of society. But of course that isn't the only option. Mothers have a right to give their babies the best food available, and to be a part of society. In countries where women are expected both to breastfeed and to be a part of the workforce the taboos are fewer.

Nevertheless we are all affected by society's expectations. If exposing your breasts embarrasses you it can also affect your milk supply. Of course you don't need to bare all. It is perfectly possible to feed a baby without being the focus of everybody else's attention. But even if the baby is discreetly tucked up under a baggy jumper you may find it hard to relax. Some of us can feed happily anywhere from a car to a committee room. Others find public feeding difficult. We need to support each others' right to feed in public if we feel happy about it or in private if we need it.

A LACTATION DIET

Junk in, junk out, as they say of computers. What we eat, and the nutrients stored in our bodies, are the sole source of supply for our babies' milk. That is why it is so important to eat well when we are breastfeeding. The elements of a good diet will be discussed later in this chapter. In addition, lactating mothers should eat:

* more calories than usual (unless you are already obviously overweight). You should get additional calories from sources such as wholemeal bread, root vegetables, rice and milk. Avoid sweet, sugary foods which provide only calories and no additional nutrients for you or your baby.
* calcium (in milk products, green vegetables and seeds), and vitamin D (from margarine and oily fish).
* A wide range of fresh vegetables and fruit (be cautious with very acidic fruits, which can upset the baby) to provide vitamins and minerals.
* Ten glasses of liquid a day from water, milk, herb teas and diluted fruit juice, etc. It is better to avoid coffee as the caffeine will go through to your baby, which may make her wakeful and jittery.

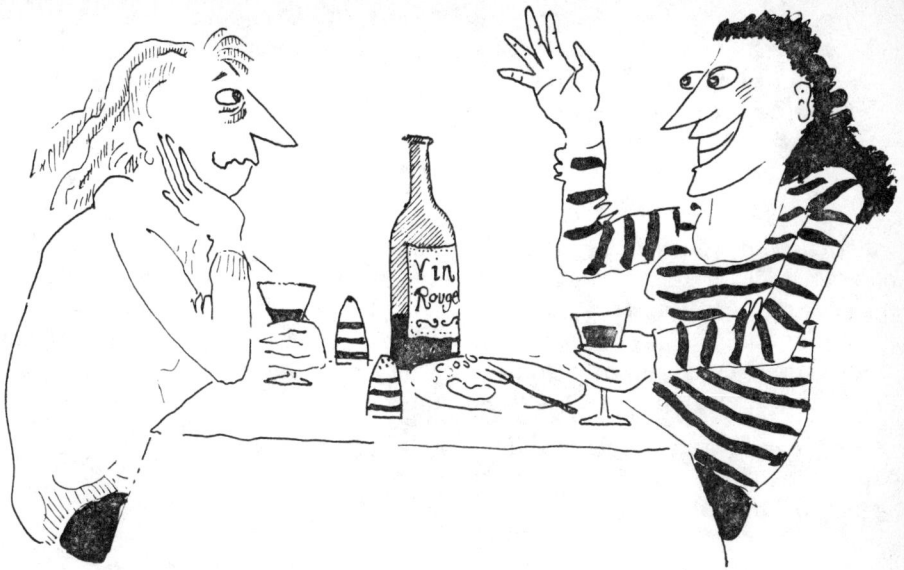

Physical difficulties

There have always been some women, in every society, who have had difficulties breastfeeding. Many of these difficulties can be solved (see p. 101),
but in a few cases even the best of good care and support will not make
the milk flow. Sadly, for many women, the frustrations of being unable to
breastfeed are compounded by guilt:

> 'I went on a breast pump every day for about ten days and got about
> half an ounce. The baby lost weight solidly for ten days. Later I found
> that I had an underactive thyroid condition, and even later still, that
> this can inhibit milk production. Most of the books I read made me
> feel guilty and a failure. It was with relief I encountered a fellow bottle-
> feeder.'

MAKING BREASTFEEDING WORK

Mothering mothers

Support from others can make all the difference in establishing successful
breastfeeding.

> 'The night she was born I had three hours' sleep. The next night she

*slept like an angel but I was so high I couldn't sleep at all. The
following evening she sucked for hours. I was exhausted but I simply
could not settle her. Finally her father came in and found me in tears.
He took her away and left me to sleep. Later he said that she lay on
his chest sucking his finger for two hours until they dozed off together.
I think that was when he fell in love with her . . . by the next evening
I had milk to feed her.'*

A partner who is sufficiently awake in the evening to take care of housework
and other kids, is probably a greater help than a half-dead one who has been
up changing nappies in the night. Women who are alone during those early
weeks may find that even post-birth euphoria is not enough to protect from
exhaustion. Friends can be a great help but not if they come for a meal, chat
all evening, and then leave the washing up:

*'I positively resent people taking up my evenings. What I long for is
someone who could just help with the work and not expect me to
entertain them.'*

Getting started

It may help to think of the first few months of a baby's life as a continuation
of pregnancy. Our bodies continue to provide everything our baby needs to
grow. Whilst they are inside us our babies are passively accepting the food
which we supply through the placenta. Once they are outside they become
an active part of the feeding process. It is the baby's suckling which regulates
the quantity of milk we produce.

The way breastfeeding is established in the first few days can make a
big difference to our success. That is why good advice is so very important.

*'She had only been at home for one night. Admittedly it was a pretty
grim night. Her baby was three days old, and the visiting midwife
suggested a bottle "to settle him so that you get a good night's sleep".
I knew that would be the beginning of the end and I offered to come
round and feed him myself if necessary rather than see her give him
a bottle so soon.'*

Giving a baby milk feeds from a bottle in the first few days can wreck any
future plans for breastfeeding. If the baby gets used to getting milk from a
teat, before she had worked out how to get it from a nipple, it can be hard
to make the transition.

For the first two or three days after birth, healthy breast-fed babies of
reasonable birth weight live mainly off the fat stored up during the last few
weeks in the womb. Breastfeeding at this time provides colostrum, which is
nourishing and full of anti-bodies, but low in calories. Real milk will not

start to come through until the third or fourth day. This is why a breastfed baby is expected to lose weight in the early days and may not regain its birth weight until it is ten days old.

Unless your baby is ill or very small there is no need for supplementary feeds at this stage, even if she appears fretful and hungry. You may have a few difficult days until your milk supply is established, but hunger will not be doing your baby any harm. (In fact, in some parts of India mothers traditionally do not feed at all until their milk comes in.) The more you allow the baby to suck, the sooner the milk will start to come. If you provide a bottle at this stage you will not only be giving unnecessary food, you will be cutting down the demands that your baby makes.

If you are having difficulty getting started it may help to spend time alone with the baby, or with an experienced helper, just to get feeding well established.

'My baby was very sleepy, I was extremely uncomfortable after the Caesarian, and I had a constant stream of visitors throughout the day. We just never really had the necessary peace and calm to work it out. If I had another baby I think I would want to restrict the visitors and spend more time on the baby.'

Sucking

The first few times you feed your baby you may be surprised to discover that it hurts. The ouch that you get as the baby starts to suck will wear off as you both get used to each other but it can be a bit of a shock at first. If this is not your first baby you may also find that suckling triggers 'after-pains'. The nipple stimulation is causing your womb to contract. This is good for your womb (it will reduce bleeding and hasten recovery after childbirth) but unpleasant. It won't last many days.

When the baby sucks she may not immediately get a mouthful of milk. The milk is lying in the glands behind the nipple but it doesn't usually come out until the baby sucks. Then you often feel a strange tingling sensation, which is your let-down reflex. Your body is telling your breasts to let the milk out. Some people hardly feel the reflex and start to pour milk as soon as the baby comes near them. Others find that it takes a good couple of minutes of suckling before the baby gets a good flow going. If you are uncomfortable or distracted your let-down reflex may be inhibited and the baby may only be getting a few drips.

'My babies have always fed best when I was alone and undisturbed and could give them my full attention. At the same time I hated to be left out of the social life around me. Most of the time my daughter fed well, cried little, and slept without fuss. On those evenings when

I had a friend around she would inevitably be crotchety, feed often, cry and on many occasions she threw up her whole feed as soon as I put her down in her cot. I am sure that, because I was not paying much attention to her, I would feed her far more than usual, she probably also gulped in more air than usual and the combination made her feel awful. I had to work out a compromise between my need for company and her need for attention.'

It is important also to make sure that the baby is 'latching on'. If she is just sucking at the end of your nipple she will not get much out. In order to suckle efficiently the baby's gums must press down on the glands behind the nipple. If your breasts are very full, or you have flat nipples, it can be more difficult for the baby to latch on efficiently. It may help to express a little milk yourself to make the breast slightly softer and then to help the baby take a big mouthful. If your baby seems unhappy, keeps snatching her head away and 'fighting' the breast you could try holding her at a different angle to see if it will help her 'latch on'.

How often and how much?

Some mothers feel very reassured by bottle feeding because the quantity is marked on the tin and you can see just how much has gone in. If your baby is content with the feeds you are giving her you have little need to worry. If she demands another in two hours you can experiment by making the next feed bigger. Far better for the baby to leave a little in the bottle than to drink the lot and still be hungry.

If you breast-feed you cannot see what is going in but if you feel confident about what you are doing, the signs are just as clear. A baby who sucks strongly from a reasonably full breast will probably get most of the feed within about ten minutes on either side. She may continue to suck and play with the nipple for pleasure after that but most of the feeding has been done. If she then burps and goes to sleep, or kicks happily for a while you will know that she had had enough. If her nappies are wet and her stools (after the first few days) soft and yellowish it is a pretty clear sign that she is getting enough.

Recent research into breastfeeding shows that the quality of milk alters not only through the months as the baby gets bigger but also through each feed. The milk produced first is called the 'fore milk'. It has a lower fat content than the 'hind milk' which comes towards the end of the feed. If your baby is just snacking several times a day, she may be getting mostly fore milk and less of the hind milk which would keep her going for longer between feeds.

This may also happen if you switch breasts before the baby has emptied

BREASTFEEDING GUIDELINES

Most problems with breastfeeding can be solved. There are a number of specialist books on the subject (see pp. 214–16) and the National Child-birth Trust and La Lèche League have counsellors who can advise you over the phone. Your local maternity hospital might also have a special-ist breastfeeding advisor and an experienced midwife can be enormously reassuring though getting a midwife who is experienced and sympath-etic with breastfeeding problems is a bit of a hit-and-miss affair.

* Make sure you are comfortable.
* Put a drink near to you so that you can sip while your baby feeds.
* Avoid very hot foods containing chillies.
* Alcohol and drugs will also go straight through to your baby. If it affects you it will affect her.
* Cracked nipples can interfere with successful feeding as well as being painful. Keep them dry and well aired and avoid breast pads and nylon bras, which trap moisture.
* Take care to empty both breasts either at the same feed or at alternate feeds. This will prevent painful engorgement (swelling), and it will also ensure that your baby is getting both the fore and hind milk.
* If you do feel a hard lump in your breast, try to unblock it by massaging the area, applying hot and cold compresses (or alternate hot and cold showers) and getting your baby to feed off that side first for a few feeds.
* If a hard, shiny, red area appears, keep feeding your baby and try to empty the breast. If you become feverish you should see a doctor as you may need antibiotics.

the first one. If you start each feed on alternate breasts and ensure that the first breast is completely emptied before switching sides (if the baby wants more), you can be sure she is getting enough of both kinds of milk. If you tend to forget which side you started with last time, try switching a ring from hand to hand to remind you, or tie a little piece of wool to your bra strap.

These days most mothers and health education 'experts' advocate 'demand' feeding. This assumes that the baby will cry when she is hungry and you will simply supply that demand by feeding her. If the two of you settle down to a reasonable pattern then this works very well. Your baby will probably want a feed every three or four hours during the day, gradually dropping feeds at night. However, some of us get into cycles of demand and supply which are harder to accommodate. Some mothers find this acceptable, others do not:

'After a slightly chaotic start I moved to feeding by the clock (not less than 3½ hours between feeds). In between I gave her a dummy which she was quite happy with. She seemed more content and satisfied after a large feed than lots of small ones.'

Increasing your supply

There will probably be times over the next few months when your baby appears to be very hungry and wants to feed all the time. If you let her suck frequently during these growth spurts, you will be giving maximum stimulation to your milk supply. That in turn will increase the supply of milk and, after a day or two, the feeding pattern will settle again. However, you must remember that you are the other side of the system. In order to make milk you need to be eating well, drinking more than usual, and getting as much rest as possible (see 'A lactation diet' below).

   If you feel your milk supply is still not sufficient, then the usual advice is to spend a couple of days relaxing completely, with your baby in bed with you, increase the calories you are consuming and drink plenty of water or fruit juice. It helps if someone else can do the cooking! Once a greater volume is being produced you should be able to return to more spaced feeds. Sometimes it is simply not possible to follow this advice.

'I suddenly realised I couldn't make that sacrifice. My other children needed me too. So I stopped trying and in two weeks he was weaned.'

Complementary bottle feeds

You may well feel pretty bad about starting bottle feeds.

'All the books say that everyone can breastfeed. They make it sound as though it's just a matter of trying harder. Everyone else in my post-natal group can do it. Why can't I? What's wrong with me?'

It is the desire to breastfeed successfully that makes us overcome obstacles in order to do it. It isn't surprising that many of us feel bad if it doesn't work. Nevertheless the decision to give your baby a bottle may take an enormous load off you. The mother quoted above was worried because her baby was gaining weight slowly (though adequately) and she found that evening feeds had become exhausting as the baby suckled almost continuously. She had no back-up from a partner who could have shared the load in the evenings and given her a break. Giving her baby a bottle, at ten weeks, was a hard decision but not one she regrets:

'If I give her a bottle at 9 pm she just lies and gurgles. Before I would be walking up and down all evening while she cried and grizzled. It has made such a difference.'

Giving complementary feeds need not be the beginning of the end of breastfeeding, as this grandmother explains:

'Normally they tell you to give a bottle after a breastfeed. I don't think this is logical. Just as we get used to regulating our intake of the first course in order to leave room for pudding, the baby will get used to taking the same amount of milk from the breast and then demand bigger and bigger bottle feeds. The logic of that is that you will very soon wean her altogether.

I had a big baby and wasn't well afterwards so I gave her a couple of ounces in a bottle at the start of the feed, and then gave the breast so that she was getting the main part of the meal from me. That way she continued to build up my supply rather than increasing the size of the bottle feeds.'

Shared feeding

Being able to share feeding with another person can give you more freedom in the early months. (See Chapter 7, 'Sharing Feeding'.) This of course is where bottle-feeders score, but it is perfectly possible for breastfeeding mothers to express their own milk using a breast pump (available in chemists) and then either leave it in the fridge (for up to one day) or freeze it for use by babysitters or your partner. However, you do have to take the same hygiene precautions as any other bottle feeder with the expressing equipment as well as the bottles.

Once breastfeeding is well established it is perfectly possible to combine breast and bottle as long as you have a regular routine. For example, you could get a partner to give a bottle every evening or at mid-day. You do not have to express milk to keep up your supply. Your body will adjust to the lower demand as long as it is regular.

BOTTLE FEEDING

What milk?

In the first year of life the Department of Health recommends that babies who are not breastfed should be fed instead on specially formulated milk which has been modified to be as close as possible to human milk. All the baby milk manufacturers provide such milks, although they vie with each other to increase their share of the market by adding new vitamins and minerals. Most manufacturers produce a range of products for young babies, middle ones and older ones, for those with allergies and for premature babies. Your doctor or health visitor should give you advice on the best formula for your particular baby.

Some babies are allergic to cow's milk, which is the basis of most formulas. This issue is discussed further under 'Allergy and food intolerance', later in this chapter. Several manufacturers are also producing something called 'follow-on' milk, which is a less modified formula invented for babies who are already on mixed feeds. These milks have no useful part to play in infant nutrition. The best bet is to go on giving your baby infant formula until she is getting the majority of her food from solids, rather than a bottle, then switch to ordinary 'doorstep' milk.

Making up feeds

It is extremely important to follow the instructions carefully when making up feeds. If you put extra formula in you will be increasing the salt content of the milk which is a) bad for your baby's kidneys and b) might make her thirsty. Formula milk looks rather thin compared to ordinary cow's milk but that is the way it is meant to be. You should never add other foods, cereals or sugar to a bottle. You will upset the very carefully balanced formula.

You must of course always use freshly boiled water to make sure that any bacteria in the water has been killed off. Cool the bottle under a running tap if necessary – do not add cool water. Once made up you can keep a whole day's worth of bottles as long as they are stored in a fridge, but don't keep a bottle that has been half-used (see Chapter 8 for more on this). You can give the baby cold milk if you like but you may prefer to warm the bottle under a hot tap. Once the milk is warm it must be given to the baby straight away and not kept.

If you want to take a bottle with you on a journey, take it out of the fridge at the last minute and put it into an insulating case (available at chemists) to keep cool, but don't leave it for more than a couple of hours.

Bottles and teats must be well cleaned before sterilising. You will need a bottle brush to scour out the inside of the bottle. Ensure that the teats are well washed inside and that no milk is clogging the hole, then rinse well and drain. Sterilising can be done with sterilising tablets (available in chemists), by boiling, steaming, or even in a microwave oven. If you use tablets, you must make sure there are no air bubbles left in the bottles (fill them up with the liquid and then submerge them) and that teats are held down under the water with a plate or lid. If you boil or steam your equipment, use a pan with a lid and boil for five minutes.

Using disposable milk bags inside a bottle cuts down the need for scrubbing and sterilising but you must still clean and sterilise the teats.

Feeding

Drip some milk from the bottle on to the back of your hand to ensure that it is not too hot. At the same time you can see whether it is coming out of the teat. Feed your baby with the bottle tilted so that the teat is always filled with milk. This will prevent her swallowing large quantities of air with her feed. If she seems frustrated and unable to get a good mouthful, the teat hole may be too small. You can add another hole with a needle sterilised in a flame. If she is flooded with milk and gasping, the hole is too big and you will need another teat.

Some parents find bottle-feeding very reassuring because the quantity is marked on the tin and you can see just how much has gone in. If your baby is content with the feeds you are giving her you have little need to worry. If she demands another in two hours you can experiment by making the next feed bigger. Far better for the baby to leave a little in the bottle than to drink the lot and still be hungry.

FROM MILK TO MUSH

Early solid feeding is rather a messy business, with as much food squidging out as going down. In the UK the usual advice is to start at four months but there is no overriding reason for this. (See 'Digestive Development', below.) It is probable that babies are physiologically ready for solids at the time their tongues are sufficiently developed to perform this task efficiently at six or seven months.

'I thought six months was good. He seemed to like any new flavour that was put in his mouth. An adventurous eater then. Now (at 8 years old) it is more difficult with new things.'

Later introduction of solids can cause difficulties. Research indicates that, even if you continue to provide most of the baby's food by breast or bottle feeding, it is wise to introduce solids in the second half of the first year so that children get used to handling food in their mouths. If feeding solids is delayed beyond twelve months, you may have some difficulty in persuading your child to eat.

'Our first boy was weaned quite early – at four months. It was quite easy. Except for celery he would eat practically anything. Our second was weaned at ten months and it wasn't so easy. There were many

things he wouldn't eat. Our last two were weaned when they were nearing their first birthday. The last one was very unpredictable with solids. A lot of patience was required.'

DIGESTIVE DEVELOPMENT

In order to make use of the food we eat our bodies need to be sufficiently mature to process it. If it starts as solid we must be able to turn it into liquid, first by chewing, then by treating it with various chemicals produced in our bodies (called enzymes) and mixing it with acids so that it can be absorbed into the bloodstream. Babies are not born with the ability to 'metabolise' every kind of food. The most obvious deficiency is lack of teeth for chewing, but the baby has a lot of maturing to do inside too.

At 35 weeks or more a healthy newborn baby will be able to suck, swallow and digest human breast milk. Few foods other than breast milk, infant formula or water, will actually be absorbed at this stage, and if you offer anything else you could trigger an allergic reaction causing stomach pain and affecting the baby's ability to absorb anything. A baby on formula will be getting all the nutrition needed from the bottle, though a little extra water (boiled and cooled) may be necessary in hot weather. A breastfed baby, providing her mother is eating well, should not even need extra water, though she may want to be fed more often when it is hot.

By four months the baby is sufficiently mature to digest some new foods, though it is not actually necessary if your baby is thriving on your milk or on formula. Sometimes big, fast-growing babies need to be fed very frequently to satisfy their appetites. In this case you may want to give them additional food. At this stage allergic reactions are less likely, although the usual medical advice is to avoid foods that are particularly likely to cause reactions such as cow's milk and cow's milk products, most grains (particularly wheat flour, which contains gluten) and eggs. These foods are better left until your baby is six months old.

By seven months your baby will have developed the mechanism with which to transfer food from the front of the tongue to the back. Before this stage food put on to a baby's tongue will only be swallowed if it is spooned right in.

How much, and what we should give our babies is a matter which often taxes the most well informed parents. Many of us get our basic advice from experts rather than our mothers or aunts. Traditional advice was consistent and modified over generations. Expert advice conflicts and seems to change by the week. This leaves us in a state of confusion and indecision. So we add

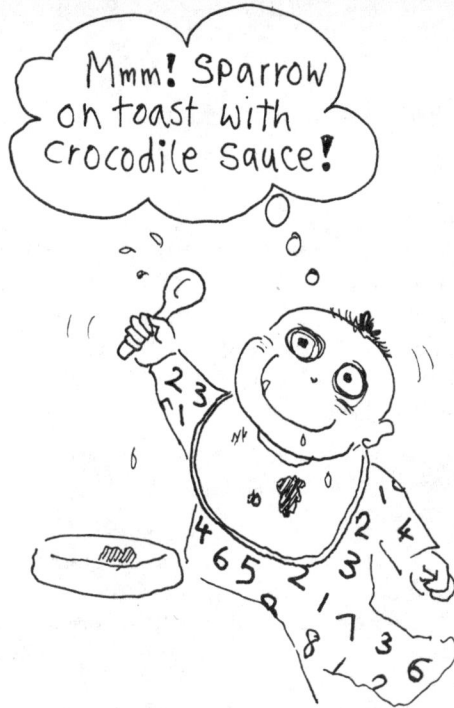

together a dash of what 'feels right' with a smattering of nutritional knowledge, and bits of what we have read in books, advertising literature, and clinic hand-outs.

'Meat was not included in the solids during the first year of introducing solids, especially red meat. We believe that giving meat so early puts an unnecessary strain on their digestive systems.'

'The first solid food I gave my daughter was a dish of mince and mash and carrots. She loved it.'

'First food was rusks. It was suggested by in-laws. I kept telling them that I didn't want to start solids too soon!'

'The first solid food I gave both my kids was baby rice, suggested by the health visitor.'

Introducing solid foods need not be a complicated business. If you leave it until the baby is old enough to reach out and grab food from the table you will probably find that curiosity will do it for you. A scrap of this and that, a teaspoonful of something else, and you will soon have a baby who is weaned on to the food you have on your table. This is the way most babies in the rest of the world go about the business of weaning. Asian dietician Kiran Shukla says:

> 'Tinned baby foods are one of my recurring fights. I always try to encourage mothers to go on with the pattern they knew back home – putting babies straight on to family foods as soon as they are off the breast.'

In Asian families following a traditional diet, the food on the table is usually prepared at home from fresh, whole products, so it is most unlikely to be harmful to an exploring child. If it is too hot, the child won't eat it, if it tastes good, he will. If, on the other hand, the family food is filled with sugar, preservatives, colourings and artificial flavourings it will not be suitable weaning food. Indeed it will not be suitable for growing human beings at all, be they large or small.

> 'Her first food was black cherry yoghurt at about three months. It was one of those occasions when Rose was hungry and Mummy was busy doing something else.'

Had this father realised what was in black cherry yoghurt he might have looked for an alternative or waited for Mummy to come home. Yoghurt is made with cow's milk and this was a fully breastfed baby who had never been introduced to cow's milk protein. Most black cherry yoghurt is coloured with Amaranth (E123), a product which has been banned in the USA, USSR, Malaysia and Sweden and restricted in several other countries. Foods which a baby is capable of eating are not necessarily foods which will do her any good.

At four months you will want to start off with simple, single foods which are very easily tolerated and unlikely to trigger an allergic reaction. The safest are: fruit (not citrus) or vegetables, rice, chicken (preferably free-range chicken to avoid the hormones which go into the feed of battery hens) or rabbit. Some children cannot manage the acidity of raw fruits, though bananas usually go down well and are very easy to mash. Other fruit can be poached in a little water. Do not add sugar or salt and make sure the food is well mashed or puréed. If your baby is over six months you can try virtually any food which can be given in a mashed-up form and does not contain additives.

> 'Mashed bananas with yoghurt was our convenience food. At meal times I would just mash up potatoes, with carrots and the odd bean. I tried putting lentils and rice through a blender but the look of it put me off so I don't suppose she felt very positive about it.'

Preparing separate meals for a baby can be exasperating, particularly in the early weeks of weaning when your baby is experimenting with tastes and textures and may well refuse to eat your carefully prepared dishes at all.

Keep in mind the fact that she is still getting most of her nutrition from your milk or formula. That milk is a perfectly balanced food. For the first few weeks, any solid food you provide is an addition to a balanced diet, so you don't have to knock yourself out making sure you get it just right and, if she doesn't eat, she can still make up the difference:

> 'Jane started solids eagerly but after the first week she started teething and simply refused to have a spoon anywhere near her mouth. I worried at first that she was going to be a faddy, difficult eater, unlike her brother, but it soon became clear that the problem was her mouth. Soon she went back to eating solid food quite happily.'

Sometimes even cooking a carrot and mashing it seems like a daunting task:

> 'Somehow I never managed to be prepared. He would be howling with hunger when I had just put the water on. By the time the carrot was cooked and cool enough to eat I had already given in and breastfed him so he was too full to be bothered with it. Worse still, I would put on the water, stick in the carrot, get sidetracked, and wind up burning the saucepan.'

While plain, home-cooked food is undoubtedly the best for your baby there can be few parents who do not occasionally turn to convenience foods. In the initial stages, between milk and meals, a few spoonfuls out of a jar or packet can save time and irritation. However, be careful what you buy. Baby foods do not contain artificial colourings and flavourings but they often contain a lot of sugar and may otherwise taste of practically nothing at all. As this mother found, children who are used to tasty food might protest:

> 'Both children ate pretty much everything I gave them. On the odd occasion I gave them baby food from a jar, they didn't like it.'

Look carefully at the labels of baby foods. Savouries now include fewer added sugars and it is possible to get pure sugar-free fruit (though it's pretty tasteless compared to a freshly stewed Cox). However, most puddings and many cereals are loaded with sugar. Be aware also that manufacturers, trying to fool wary parents, now add many different sugars including glucose, fructose, invert syrup, maltose, and even caramel. These are no better for your children than old-fashioned sucrose (sugar). If you are concerned about giving your baby milk or gluten you should check labels carefully. Many powdered foods have dried milk powder in them.

If you have a freezer you need never resort to jars and packets. You can simply cook up a variety of vegetables and fruit, put them through a blender, and freeze them in ice cube trays. You can then heat them up as you need them. However, don't freeze meat- or fish-based dishes this way. These foods must be heated to boiling point for a few minutes before serving (see Chapter

8) and, if you are only using small amounts, it is very hard not to burn them.

FROM GLOOP TO LUMPS

In the second half of its first year your baby will probably begin to acquire teeth. However, a couple of front teeth can be less than helpful. They may be good at biting things off but, without back teeth to grind the bits up, they are not much help nutritionally. At this stage you need to be particularly careful about the kind of food you give your baby. A carrot may be satisfying for a teething baby to chew on, but if a bit is accidentally bitten off, she may choke on it. Soft fruits (with stones removed) should be no problem and bread crusts are satisfying gum-rubbers and tend to disintegrate when they get wet, which is safer.

'On holiday in California, our baby was always given a bagel on a ribbon when we went out to eat. He loved it.'

Experience at chewing, even before teeth appear, will accustom your baby to the idea of eating something in a solid form and make gums strong. Babies who don't learn to use their gums can become young children who don't want to use their teeth. The move from sloppy food to stiffer, roughly mashed food and gradually to lumpy food is a matter for experiment. Even before teeth come through the gums become hard enough to 'chew' soft, but relatively lumpy food such as bananas, pieces of cooked potato, bread and small pieces of fish or chicken. Meat is harder and is better minced or cut up very fine.

A baby who has no back teeth to grind with cannot easily digest foods with a tough outer skin such as lentils, beans, raisins and seeds unless they are ground up. As any nappy changer will note, most of these things go straight through, whole, until an age when the child not only has back teeth but is prepared to use them properly. Avoid giving nuts (unless they are ground up) and in particular peanuts, which can get stuck in the baby's windpipe and are very dangerous.

In small amounts undigested food will not matter much, but nor will it do any good. It is no use giving a small child a spoonful of sesame seeds in order to boost her calcium intake. She will be unable to break down the seeds and all the calcium will end up in her nappy. Make sure that these high fibre foods don't fill her up with indigestible material and leave insufficient room for nutrients that she can use for energy. It is possible for a child to become seriously undernourished if she is unable to make use of a high proportion of her diet.

FROM MILK TO MIXED

Let your child guide you as to how fast you move from a milk-based diet to a mixed diet. In the first six months milk should predominate. In the second half of the year, milk may gradually give way to solid food and become merely another drink. Once the balance has moved from occasional solid snacks to a solid-food-based diet you will need to pay much more attention to what your child eats.

While milk is still the major part of the diet you should stick to breast milk or infant formula because it contains all the vitamins and minerals needed in the right balance of protein and carbohydrate. Once your baby is eating three hearty meals a day containing a balance of nutrients (see below), you can move to doorstep milk in a cup or beaker. Pasteurised milk need not be boiled as long as it is not left open in a warm room (see Chapter 8). A pint of milk, or the equivalent in yoghurt and cheese (¼ lb of cheese = 1 pint of milk), is the recommended daily amount for a young child.

Once solid food is an established part of her diet, start introducing some drinks in a beaker too. If you use the kind with a lid and spout you should find that by the fifth month she will be very keen to help herself and, by time solid foods predominate, she can handle her own cup and drink what she needs.

A GOOD DIET

Vegetables and fruit

These should be the basis of any good diet. If your children get a mixture of green, yellow and white vegetables through the week, and some raw fruit or salad every day, they will be getting most of the vitamins and minerals they need.

*'In Spain even the poorest families know that children should have
something raw every day. If they cannot afford fruit then their
children will get tomatoes with their meal.'*

Cereals, bread and potatoes

These should provide most of your child's need for energy. A hungry child can fill up on bread, rice, pasta or potatoes. Since these are the basic foods for virtually every diet in the world the quality of the cereals you eat are very important. They lay down the basis of your child's daily diet. Bread should be *wholemeal* right from the very start. The white soggy stuff which passes for bread in Britain is stripped of most of its vitamins, minerals and fibre. Those added back do not compensate for what is taken out. Breakfast cereals should also be made from whole grain without added sugar (for example Puffed Wheat) or with only very small quantity of added sugar (for example Shreddies). There is no need to add sugar at the table.

Protein foods

These are the body-building foods but they also provide a range of vitamins and minerals and slow down the release of energy so that other foods are used more efficiently. Meat, poultry, fish, eggs and dairy products (cheese, milk and yoghurt) are the major protein sources. However, combinations of beans with cereals in forms such as dal and rice, pitta bread and humous or even beans on toast provide a good source of protein which is cheap. Include some protein (not always meat, which also has a high saturated fat content) in every main meal.

Essential Fatty Acids (EFAs)

These play an important part in the absorption of vitamins. They affect brain development and the functioning of the nervous system. These EFAs are found in most liquid vegetable oils (particularly sunflower and corn oil), in fresh vegetables and in fish. Most nutritionists recommend that animal fats (other than dairy products) should be eaten in moderation as they may lay down the basis for heart disease in adulthood.

Fibre

This is present in most unprocessed foods (other than milk products). It helps the digestive system to work properly. Insufficient fibre is associated with a whole number of the so-called diseases of civilisation from heart disease to bowel cancer. If you are using whole foods there will be sufficient fibre in your child's diet, and it is unnecessary to add any more.

Liquid

This is also an important part of the diet. The best drink is water. During the first year water should always be boiled. You can boil a bottleful in the morning and keep it in a fridge. Add some fruit juice to the water if your

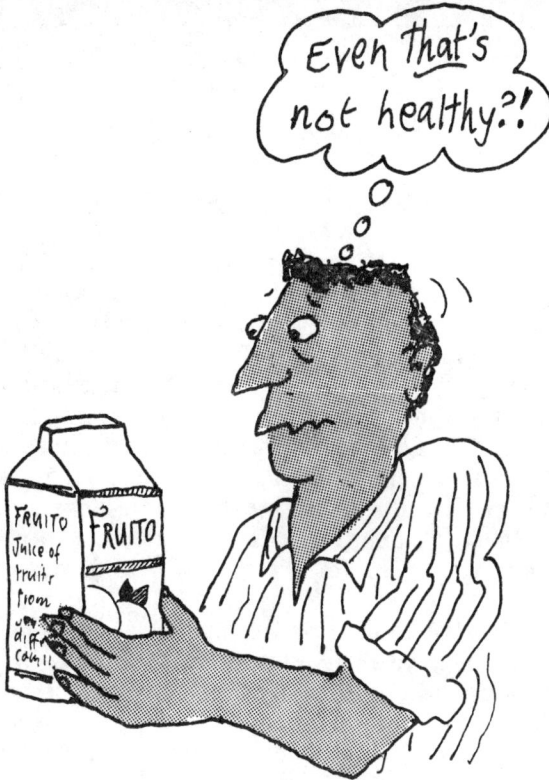

children demand more taste but don't give pure fruit juice undiluted as it is a concentrated food with a very high level of natural sugar and the acidity is hard on the teeth. You can try cooled herb teas, avoiding the prepared kinds which are heavily sugared. You can buy herb teas in health food shops and chemists and prepare them yourself. Herbs also have medicinal properties, so ask for advice before you buy. Avoid ordinary tea and coffee which contain tannin and caffeine.

Some important foods

These contain specific minerals and vitamins that children need for growth: egg yolks, liver, pulses or dried fruit, all of which contain iron (breast milk does not contain much iron); milk, crushed seeds or plenty of green vegetables, which contain calcium. During the first year at least, egg yolks should be *hard* boiled to kill any bacteria.

WHAT CHILDREN DO NOT NEED

Refined sugar

This is a highly concentrated food which contains nothing of value other than calories.

Children need calories for energy but they can get it from other foods which also provide vitamins, minerals and fibre and contribute to the general balance of their diet rather than overbalancing it in the direction of energy (which may simply be converted to fat).

Pure sugar will rot their teeth, rob their bodies of vitamins needed for other things, stop them from enjoying other tastes and above all, ruin their appetites for the kinds of food which they need to grow and stay healthy. It is also habit-forming. We all start out with quite a 'sweet tooth' (breast milk is very sweet) but, unless we are weaned off it, sweet tastes and high energy foods will continue to dominate our diets, pushing out the more important foods and undermining our health.

When a child is ill or recovering from an illness, and has very little appetite, there may be a case for giving sugar or glucose in liquid form (such as rehydrating solutions discussed in Chapter 8), because it is very easily absorbed. At other times, refined, added sugars from any source (concentrated fruit juice, glucose, maltose and so on) are best avoided, or used in moderation.

Experiment with recipes which allow you to lower the amount of sugar you use. If you sweeten foods do so sparingly – half a teaspoon of honey will usually be quite sufficient to sweeten a small bowl of plain yoghurt. Those little pots of fruit-flavoured yoghurt contain as much as three teaspoons of sugar. It is also added to many manufactured foods such as baked beans. Sweets are made entirely of sugar and most fizzy drinks have a very high sugar content too. As far as possible try to avoid foods where sugar is already added and you have no control over how much has been used.

Additives

Colourings, flavourings and preservatives are used in many foods eaten by children: fruit squash and fizzy drinks, yoghurts, cake mixes and desserts. Few of these chemicals have been proved to be safe and many are known to cause side effects, from rashes to behavioural problems, particularly in children (see Allergy and food intolerance, later in this

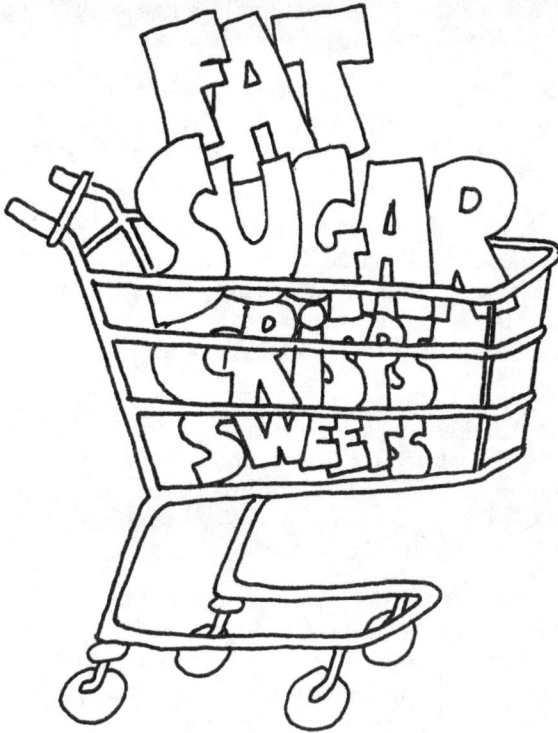

chapter.) Drinks can be particularly bad. Cola and Lucozade contain caffeine, the substance that gives coffee its kick. Many orange-coloured drinks contain Tartrazine. Tartrazine and caffeine can both cause irritable, jittery behaviour and sleep problems. According to food writer Geoffrey Cannon, the average child in Britain will have consumed as much as half a pound of dyes by the age of twelve. Try to avoid foods with additives of any kind. If you need to use them, do so sparingly.

GOOD HABITS START YOUNG

British people eat what is probably one of the worst diets in the world. We also have more heart disease, more children with the disease spina bifida, and worse teeth than other countries and we come out badly on a host of other indices of health. Many experts feel that our diet is a major reason for these problems. We have the highest consumption of sweets and chocolates in Europe and the lowest consumption of green vegetables and fruit. Look at the average supermarket trolley and you will see that it is loaded with manufactured foods filled with chemical additives. The following diets are fairly typical of what young British children eat:

Breakfast: Sunshine Orange Breakfast, water, milk.
Lunch: Autumn Vegetable Casserole, water, rusk, milk.
Supper: chocolate bar followed by cow's milk with a teaspoon of sugar at bedtime.

This diet, taken from a survey on Sugar in Baby Foods published by the Maternity Alliance (Lyn Durwood Health Education Council, 1988) contains added sugars at every meal. Doorstep milk was the only unprocessed food. There were no fresh vegetables or fruit.

The Bristol Child Development Programme came up with the typical diet of a toddler in Scotland:

Breakfast: cornflakes, milk, cup of tea.
Mid morning: chocolate cream egg, chocolate bar.
Lunch: baked potato, slice of white bread and butter.
Afternoon: ice cream, two slices of cake, two digestive biscuits.
Evening: chips, two slices of white bread and butter, cup of coffee.

Once again, sugary foods dominate, alongside refined flour (white bread, cake and biscuits), which is almost as low in nutrients. Giving tea and coffee to children is simply feeding them stimulants (how many two-year-olds need stimulating?). A report in *The Guardian* (4 April, 1986) about a survey of school children's diets showed that things do not improve. They lived largely on crisps, chips and biscuits.

Geoffrey Cannon, author of *The Politics of Food* (Century, 1988), interviewed Walter Barker, head of the child development programme, about these findings and he said:

'The brain is still developing in the first two years of life. Most of the children from poor households, and many of the children from better-off households, were eating a poor diet, high in sugars and low in whole foods. This can lead to retarded brain growth after weaning. The children will never reach their full potential.'

Good eating is not simply a matter of knowledge or even of income. As this mother living in Liverpool pointed out:

'I bought an iron casserole for her meals but it was a challenge to find fresh vegetables and fish in our area.'

While on maternity leave, searching for fresh food may be a challenge but, as the same mother found, priorities can shift when you return to work:

'Once I started working full time I no longer had the energy to prevent the rest of the family going for quick answers to a hungry child coming

home from nursery at six o'clock. By the time she gets home she is
famished and it is too easy to start giving her snacks in the car. In
fact the car is littered with crisp and sweet wrappings and she has
lived almost exclusively on fish fingers, sausages and chips since she
was about a year old.'

Busy lives and lack of available fresh food make providing a good diet much
harder than it should be. As supermarkets put small shops out of business,
fresh food is less accessible than ever for those of us who do not have
access to good transport facilities, or the time to make lengthy trips to
supermarkets. If you do not have a local supply of fresh vegetables and fruit
you have to make compromises. Here are some suggestions:

• Potatoes are available everywhere and they can be stored. They are a
very good source of carbohydrate, fibre and vitamins. For many people they
are the major source of vitamin C. Baked potatoes are easy to prepare and,
with added beans, cheese or yoghurt, provide a good healthy meal.
• Eat soft fruit, which doesn't keep, at the start of the week but keep apples,
pears and bananas for the later days.
• Be sure to eat fresh vegetables at the weekend and then use frozen ones
towards the end of the week when supplies run out. Frozen vegetables have
a higher vitamin content than limp ones stored for too long.
• Give your children something uncooked every day. Apples and carrots can
be grated for younger children; sliced and peeled cucumber is easy for most
children to manage.
• Avoid reheating cooked vegetables or peeling and soaking them in
advance as the vitamin content will drop. If you use frozen vegetables, reheat
to boiling point and then serve them. They do not need to be re-cooked.
• Cook in iron saucepans which will provide added iron.
• If you are late home and your child is hungry, give her a plate full of raw
carrot, apple slices and a handful of raisins; some cheese and a couple of
slices of bread or some pasta is just as quick to cook as sausages and far
more nutritious.

'When I come back late and I'm too tired to cook, we have a picnic on
the living-room floor with all her dollies and then she has even been
known to eat wholemeal bread and yoghurt!'

• If you regularly provide sausages and fish fingers make sure your children
also eat freshly cooked or raw vegetables and fruit – not just chips.
• grow your own bean sprouts (better still, get your children to grow them).
This provides a source of vitamins, minerals and protein which is absolutely
fresh, accessible and cheap.
• Don't let your children make too many choices if you take them shopping.
They will go for foods in highly coloured wrappings just as the manufacturers
and designers intended. Most are loaded with sugar and colouring. If you

explain why you are making these choices they will be learning something about food too.

INSTITUTIONAL FOODS

'I have only felt in control of Rosie's diet during the period when I was not in full-time work. She started having the odd crisp and fizzy drink at her first nursery as a treat. Her permanent nursery tried whole foods but has now slipped back into providing a lot of baked beans. When you are working it actually lessens your confidence as a parent. The sense of being unable to control some of the most important things can be devastating.'

If you are working full time, the last thing you feel like doing is taking on the nursery or school over the provision of nutritious meals, yet a good food policy can be a godsend to busy parents:

'It is such a relief not to have to worry about food during the week. I can give her yoghurt and fruit, or a peanut butter sandwich, and an apple, with a glass of milk because I know that at lunch time she has been filled up with high quality food.'

Many education authorities have adopted a good food policy and now provide a higher proportion of whole foods, salads and fruit. It is well worth lobbying those that do not. You can write to local councillors, approach the parent governors in your school or bring the subject up at the Parent-Teachers Association. It may be more difficult to have an impact on a private nursery, and trying to explain your eating habits to your childminder may seem difficult because it may feel like a criticism of the way she feeds her family. However, it is better to be clear about what you want than to suffer in silence. This childminder says:

'Get all your problems out into the air. It is your child and you are paying her to do a job for you.'

FADDY CHILDREN

Children may themselves conspire to make it virtually impossible to feed them properly.

'By nine months he was eating fish, meat, pulses, fruit, vegetables, cheese, yoghurt, pasta – you name it. This continued until he was eighteen months old and then he suddenly stopped eating. Literally seemed to go off everything and since then mealtimes have been a battlefield.'

'I have sat and cried over my children not eating and had row after row at the table, but I don't bother any more. They do not seem to be under-nourished and don't get any more illness than other children.'

Food fads are extremely common and can cause enormous tension. Sometimes a child has simply 'gone off' a particular food and, if left alone, will probably change back again in time. Peggy Wynn, a grandmother and nutrition writer, has this to say:

'Respect all refusals – the child has a feel for what he needs. No greens one day, double helping the next will mean he feels like them.'

She recognises also the need for occasional subterfuge to get a child in a faddy stage to eat food that she needs.

'I find that children won't eat liver if you give it to them plain. I always get a few ounces put in with my mince and then they don't notice it.'

There can be many reasons why a child doesn't like something. The texture of the food may be as important as the taste. I remember loathing spaghetti as a child because I didn't like the feel of it. Many children become deeply suspicious of mixed-up foods. A child who refuses a chicken casserole may happily eat chicken, potatoes and carrots if they are supplied separately.

Fear that a child is not eating enough to keep a bird alive can lead you into providing food which, in your heart, you know is not good for him.

'My son loves his food, my daughter eats hardly anything – half a slice of toast, half a sandwich, small meals. She loves McDonalds and chips but so long as she eats something that is better than nothing.'

While it is sensible to make small compromises, it is fatal if you give in entirely to your children's fads and allow them to use meal times to manipulate you. Anne Kilby is Paediatrician in a London hospital.

'So many parents get anxious because the child doesn't eat at meal times and then they give a snack to make up for it. So then the child won't eat the next meal either. If you add up the snacks they have eaten during the day, it turns out to be quite a lot. They are just not eating meals. The only way to cope with fads is to be calm about them. Children do not starve themselves.'

If you only ever provide food which is reasonably nutritious you need not worry if your child stops eating most things. Even a very narrow range of food will probably provide most of his needs in the short term:

'He now will not eat any meat, very little in the way of vegetables, no fish or pulses, occasionally spaghetti, some bread, some cheese, fruit is OK and lots of yoghurt.'

This mother worries about her child's eating and yet, compared to children in the Bristol survey, this is a pretty good diet. It shows that even when a child restricts what he is prepared to eat, as long as the food you provide is good food, he will eat a reasonably balanced diet. I personally believe its a good idea to go on offering a wide range of foods. These parents insist on their son eating just a tiny bit of everything.

'I try not to be too anxious. I insist on him having a bit of everything that goes on the table. That can create problems but I don't ask him to have enormous quantities, only a bit of things he hates. I find that, after a while, he starts to like the things that he hated.'

Other parents find that insisting on eating even a little of unliked foods creates a battleground and makes meals a misery. It may be enough to put food on the table, or a little on the plate, without insisting that they eat it:

'It is very important not to make too big an issue of it or he will dig his heels in and refuse it. I try to make it feel as though he has made a positive discovery on his own when, after disliking something for a while, he finds that it tastes nice again. I always say that I am putting some on his plate just in case he has changed his mind since last time. Then I try to ignore it.'

Living in an advanced Western country our children are most unlikely to starve, and yet we still tend to respond to our child's need for food with instant gratification. If you really think your child is particularly hungry you can give her pieces of carrot or a cup of milk, or just bring forward supper by half an hour. If you give into the demands for sugary snacks you will be supplying calories for the moment in place of a longterm good health. If your child is already hooked on a small range of 'junk' foods you may need help in changing his diet, but don't be afraid he will go hungry. Even if he refuses to eat at all for a couple of days it will do less longterm harm than a continuing diet of sugar and white flour. Children do respond to clear food rules as long as they are not accompanied by threats or wheedling.

'We don't allow any snacks in the crèche. The children get fruit juice at 10.15 and then lunch at about 12.20. Some of them do get tired and hungry and occasionally a child gets too tired to eat and then wakes up in a real temper. We will compromise by giving some children milk instead of fruit juice if their parents want it but everyone agrees that the pleasure of seeing them tuck away platefuls of pasta, vegetables and rice is worth the sacrifice of the occasional hunger pang.'

Sometimes a child who will eat virtually nothing at home is prepared to try anything when eating in company. One child in our crèche who was famed for eating three or four platefuls of anything in front of him went through a period of refusing virtually anything but pasta at home. Children may also differ in the time they take over eating. While one will wolf the whole lot down in minutes, another will sit over a meal for an hour.

'I try to be patient. If everyone leaves the table, she will get up too even if she hasn't eaten enough. I am also strict about not providing pudding until everyone has finished the first course. If she sees her brother with an apple she won't finish her vegetables.'

A demand for food is not always connected with hunger. It is just as likely to be a demand for attention. If you have a friend around to visit in the afternoon you can be sure that your child will come in with a constant stream of demands for food and drink. Mostly she is trying to win back some of your attention. These sorts of issues are discussed in Chapter 3. However, if you have food rules it is worth sticking to them, otherwise your child is learning that when guests come she can eat what she likes.

ALLERGY AND FOOD INTOLERANCE

There is a great deal of truth in the old adage that 'one man's meat is another man's poison.' Foods which to most of us are a vital source of healthy nourishment are, to a minority, a major source of misery, causing anything from skin rashes or eczema, to fits of screaming and broken nights. However, a great deal of misinformation circulates about allergies within the medical profession and amongst parents too. The parents who put down every sneeze and snuffle to a food intolerance do exist but they are probably no more common, and a lot less of a problem, than the doctors who refuse to credit the possibility of allergy or intolerance at all. As this mother of two milk-intolerant children said:

'There is something about being a reasonably intelligent woman which sets off alarm bells for them. They just say "Have you been reading something? Don't get excited about it." They seem to feel that you shouldn't try to find out about things that might affect your children's health.'

So just how worried should we be about the effects of certain foods and additives?

Preventing allergies

Nobody wants their child to be unhappy, undernourished or in pain. If a baby eats something to which she or he is truly allergic or intolerant these are the likely symptoms. It is for this reason that it makes sense to keep babies off foods which are likely to cause a reaction (see 'From milk to mush',

p. 105). Some food researchers also believe that by avoiding these foods in the first four to six months, and waiting until the digestive system has matured a little, babies are less likely to develop allergies in later childhood. However, according to paediatrician Anne Kilby:

'There is no clear answer about whether avoidance of cow's milk and other allergens in the first six months will reduce the likelihood of allergy in later childhood. Most children who are allergic to cow's milk grow out of it by the age of two and a half or three, but they might still go on to have other allergies later.'

Nevertheless, like many other parents, Dr Kilby kept her first two children off cow's milk, gluten (in wheat-based products) and eggs until they were six months old. So while excluding allergens in the early months may not be the longterm health insurance policy that people hoped, it is probably still worth trying to avoid them, particularly if you have a strong family history of allergy (eczema, asthma, hay fever, skin rashes, etc.).

In the early stages of weaning a breastfed baby will not need a very wide range of additional foods and so it is relatively simple to exclude the foods most commonly associated with allergy. However, even this might not be enough if your child is allergic to cow's milk. In some documented cases breastfed babies have developed allergies because of cow's milk consumed by their mothers, which in rare cases gets through into the breast milk.

This does not mean that all mothers should stop eating dairy products. For the vast majority of us, these foods are an important source of calories and the calcium that we need to replenish our supplies. Normally we have the necessary enzymes to break down cow's milk protein efficiently and it should not get through, in that form, to our own milk. However, for those few mothers and babies where there is a real problem it may be necessary for the mother to give up these foods too. This mother had already had one child with a diagnosed milk allergy:

'Dominic had colic. We saw the paediatrician who had originally seen my first child, Emma. He had initially been sceptical about the milk allergy but, seeing that a milk-free diet had worked with her, he advised me to cut all lactose (dairy products) out of my own diet for six months while I was breastfeeding. It certainly helped. The persistent all-day screaming stopped and she just cried in the evenings.'

For bottle-fed babies there is an immediate difficulty. Most formulas are based on the food most likely to cause intolerance or allergy. This a major cause of worry for many bottle-feeding mothers:

'GUILT GUILT GUILT. The baby's health becomes a worry because you think you have failed.'

It is likely, however, that if a baby is going to be cow's-milk sensitive there will be some reaction pretty quickly, in which case it would be sensible to turn to a soy-based formula. Turning to soy products might not solve all your problems. Children given large quantities of soy-based products may develop an intolerance to them too (and there is some concern about the level of aluminium in soy milk products). In such cases, your doctor can prescribe a specially prepared infant formula.

Between six months and a year you can start introducing suspect foods slowly, one at a time. If your child reacts badly, then leave that food out for a while and try again. While it is sensible to avoid the additives for ever if you can, it is not worthwhile cutting out wheat, milk and eggs in the long term unless there is a very clear indication that they are causing trouble, or they do not form a major component of your household diet. For those eating a traditional European diet, milk, wheat and eggs are staple foods and it is hard to avoid them without upsetting the balance of the diet, as this family discovered:

> 'We give her soya milk on cereal, white fish and a white bread roll every day to provide calcium. Fortunately we have just discovered soya ice-cream, which she loves, but it is really very difficult. We used to be vegetarians, but since we can no longer eat cheese we have found that we have to include chicken in our diet just to make sure she has enough protein.'

Even if a child is allergic to one or more of these foods, it is worth trying to introduce them again every six months or so as the allergy will often disappear as the digestive system matures.

Spotting an allergy

Some allergies announce themselves with absolute clarity:

> 'Janie gets a rash on her face (even now at 11 years old) if she eats red/orange food colourings (E102 or E110).

> 'At one time my daughter could not eat eggs. Her skin used to break out all red/pink.'

> 'I breast fed and as soon as I mixed even a tiny bit of cow's milk with her cereal she got a rash all round her chin and face.'

Clearly recognised childhood illnesses such as asthma or eczema may also be triggered by allergies to food, pollen, house dust and animal fur. These allergies are usually treated with drugs but can also respond to dietary changes:

> 'One child developed eczema shortly after starting in our crêche. After

about eighteen months it became much more severe and the itching and scratching set up a nasty patch of inflamed and infected skin on his arms. He was miserable and angry if any child so much as touched his sore arm. His mother asked us if we would be prepared to help her put him on a milk-free diet. Since food was prepared by five different parents each week this required some thought by all of us but everyone agreed that it was worth a try. His skin cleared rapidly (though not completely) and he has been a great deal happier since.'

Cow's milk intolerance is much more common amongst African and Asian families, who do not traditionally eat dairy products.

FOODS WITH A STRONG ASSOCIATION WITH ALLERGY

Cow's milk
This covers all dairy products including most margarines, which contain whey. Goat's milk is close in composition to cow's milk and may also cause a reaction (it should be boiled as it is not sold in a pasteurised form). Soy products are a useful alternative but may also cause reactions in some children. Cheese and yoghurt made from sheep's milk are usually tolerated.

Gluten
This is found in wheat, barley, rye and to some extent in oats, and it cannot be tolerated by some babies. If a baby with coeliac disease (as it is called) eats gluten, the result is diarrhoea, often pain and general failure to thrive. There is some evidence that if gluten is excluded from the diet for four to six months, the risk of developing the disease is reduced. Baby foods which are gluten-free will usually be labelled. If the foods do not specify 'gluten free' they are best avoided. Rice is the safest cereal to give to a baby and it is the first weaning food in many countries all over the world. Oat cereals are pretty well tolerated.

Eggs
These can cause skin rashes, and they were found to be a problem in children suffering from eczema, migraine and behavioural disturbance. It is usually recommended that only the yolk of the egg should be given to babies between six months and one year. After that, whole eggs can be introduced.

Chocolate
This comes high on the list of sensitive foods for most allergic conditions, in particular migraine.

Fish
An allergy to fish may cause urticaria (localised skin rashes).

Oranges and grapes
These have been implicated in studies of allergy. It is wise to avoid them in the early introduction of solids.

Additives

Food additives can cause a wide range of allergic reactions and they are certainly implicated in hyperactivity and migraine. The best bet is to avoid all of them, but this is a list of the ones which are known to have harmful effects in some people. All artificial additives are banned in foods marketed specifically for babies and infants. Foods with E numbers are allowed for export to all EEC countries. Those that do not have E numbers have been banned in some countries and are not approved by the EEC.

Avoid these additives

Colourings
Coal tar dyes: Chocolate Brown (HT); tartrazine, yellow (E102); Sunset yellow (E110), Amaranth, red (E123), Ponceau 4R, red (E124), Brilliant Blue FCF (133) (this colouring has been banned by a number of expert committees on food colourings but has subsequently been allowed back on to the market). Any food with a blue colouring should be considered suspect.
    Natural colouring: Annatto, yellow, orange (E160b).

Preservatives
Benzoic Acid and Benzoates (E210 and E219); Sulphur Dioxide and Sulphites (E220–227); Nitrates and Nitrites (E249-E252).

Flavour enhancer
Monosodium Glutamate and Gluamates (621–623)

Antioxidants
BHA and BHT (E320 and E321)

Other symptoms of allergy may be overlooked or assumed to be 'behavioural problems' as these two mothers found:

'Emma was a very active baby but well, lively and gaining weight normally. At five months I started her on solids. She started losing weight, and took to waking up all through the night screaming with pain. I took her off milk and she did seem to improve a little but the doctor persuaded me to put her back on. They said there was no reason to suppose she had a milk allergy. By the time she was one year old she was still not gaining weight properly, she had loose stools five times a day and she wasn't sleeping well. We decided to try taking her off milk again. Within ten days she was happier, sleeping better and, within a month, had started to gain weight.'

This child, at two and a half, is still off milk in spite of many attempts to reintroduce it. Her parents find that each time she eats so much as a cream cake she will be up in the night with stomach pains. Her problem is that the milk cannot be broken down properly and her gut lining becomes increasingly damaged, which in turn prevents the absorption of other foods. The result: low weight gain, diarrhoea, stomach pain and an unhappy child. The difficulty with an intolerance is that the reaction is not always immediate so doctors may find it hard to spot.

Migraine can also be triggered by allergens. Since small children cannot describe what they are feeling, a headache may be mis-diagnosed as hunger, a tummy ache, or just 'bad temper'.

'There was no recognisable sign of allergy such as a rash, diarrhoea, or asthma. At fourteen months old he just started having temper tantrums which got worse and worse. I was convinced he had a brain tumour. After a sleep he would scream and scream and we could never be sure what sort of mood he would wake up in. Between three and four he started getting both asthma and eczema. Still nobody suspected food as the problem. He was still having these terrible fits of screaming at seven and eight years old and I was desperate. I heard about additive allergies and took him off all additives. That didn't help. Then I decided to try cutting out milk. I had just qualified as a Health Visitor and I think I had begun to hear about milk allergy. Within three days he was a different child. He has never had another screaming fit.'

Few doctors would recognise this as a milk allergy because it doesn't fit into the accepted medical description of allergy. Nevertheless, in a study of childhood migraine (Eggar, 1985) more children were found to be sensitive to cow's milk than any other single food, and cow's milk is also implicated in studies of hyper-activity (children who are over-active). So clearly milk can affect behaviour in some sensitive children.

Most of the allergy or intolerance described here was associated with milk, but in a strictly controlled trial, carried out by doctors at Great Ormond Street Hospital (Eggar, 1985), colourings and preservatives were found to be even more closely associated with behavioural disturbance.

'Colourants (Tartrazine) and preservatives (Benzoates) were the commonest substances that provoked abnormal behaviour in our patients, although no patient in our series reacted to them alone.'

Cow's milk was the second most common allergen and a high proportion of those allergic to milk also reacted to soya. Other foods which came high on the list were: chocolate, grapes, wheat, oranges, eggs and peanuts. Since these were a group of children with severe problems and multiple allergies, a large number of other foods also caused reactions for some of them.

Coping with an allergy

While these substances can be responsible for a wide range of symptoms it is important to be sure of cause and effect before making changes to your child's diet which could limit his or her diet unnecessarily. Not every child who sleeps badly has a tummy ache (see Chapter 4), and a child who is unsettled or has temper tantrums may simply be going through a normal developmental stage (see 'Angry children' in Chapter 3). If you do want to look at the effect of eliminating foods do so carefully.

Obviously stopping all juices with colourings can only be of benefit, but cutting out milk may cause problems. You will have to find ways of replacing calcium, protein, vitamin A and the fats which are important in the diet of a young child. It may help to learn about the diets of people who do not normally eat dairy products (such as the Chinese) to get an idea of how to balance a milk-free diet.

Don't drop more than one food at a time and make sure that you try the change for at least two weeks, keeping a diary of sleep, behaviour, eating, stools, etc. to give yourself an objective measurement of change. If you suspect more than one food intolerance try to get a referral to a paediatrician. However, don't expect anybody to take you very seriously at first. Many doctors are deeply suspicious of parents who believe that their children's behaviour is caused by allergy.

For many parents, the sheer effort involved in changing a child's diet is worse than coping with the effects of a mild allergy. This family has allergy on both sides: asthma and urticaria (a skin rash). Both the daughters suffer from ear infections, one has eczema, and the other has asthma:

'I was very careful not to give them dairy products or gluten before six months and that may be why Rosie's asthma did not start until she was six. She has never had a severe attack and the treatment controls the condition very quickly. Jane's eczema has never been bad enough for me to take on the problem of cutting all dairy products out of her diet. I know how hard it would be so, at the moment, on balance, I prefer to stick with medical treatment for the condition and let them eat the things they like.'

Chapter 6

WHAT COMES OUT

What comes out of a child is almost as important as what goes in. From a positive point of view it tells us quite a lot about our children's health. However it is also a major expense (generating a whole industry in products invented to help parents cope); a source of friction; and often an emotional minefield. There is not much you can do about the cost of nappies (buying disposables is not significantly cheaper than washing terries), but a straight-forward and relatively relaxed approach to the whole business of poo and pee should help you to approach the toilet training phase with equanimity.

WHAT TO EXPECT FROM YOUR BABY

The first six months

I knew when my baby had last had a shit. As the paediatrician checked him over, he squirted it all down his white coat. When we arrived home a couple of hours later I changed his nappy and it was dirty again . . . Panic! I had only had him home five minutes and I was convinced that he was already suffering from a life-threatening attack of diarrhoea. I began to think that I should never have left the safety of the hospital.

I need not have panicked. A healthy baby who is feeding well should wet at least a dozen nappies a day. Dirty nappies are far more erratic. A newborn, breastfed baby can dirty half a dozen nappies a day or only one or two a week. Bottle-fed babies should produce at least one dirty nappy a day. Gradually they will settle down to about one or two every day or two for breastfed babies and one or two a day for bottle-fed babies.

In the first two or three days after birth babies produce a sticky black stuff called meconium. As your milk comes in it will gradually turn green and then bright yellow. If you are bottle feeding it will be a lighter yellow or light brown and slightly bulkier than the soupy consistency of a breast-fed baby's stools. Although the 'sour milk' smell of baby shit is not to every-one's taste it should not really be unpleasant.

Some babies find passing stools quite hard work in the early weeks.

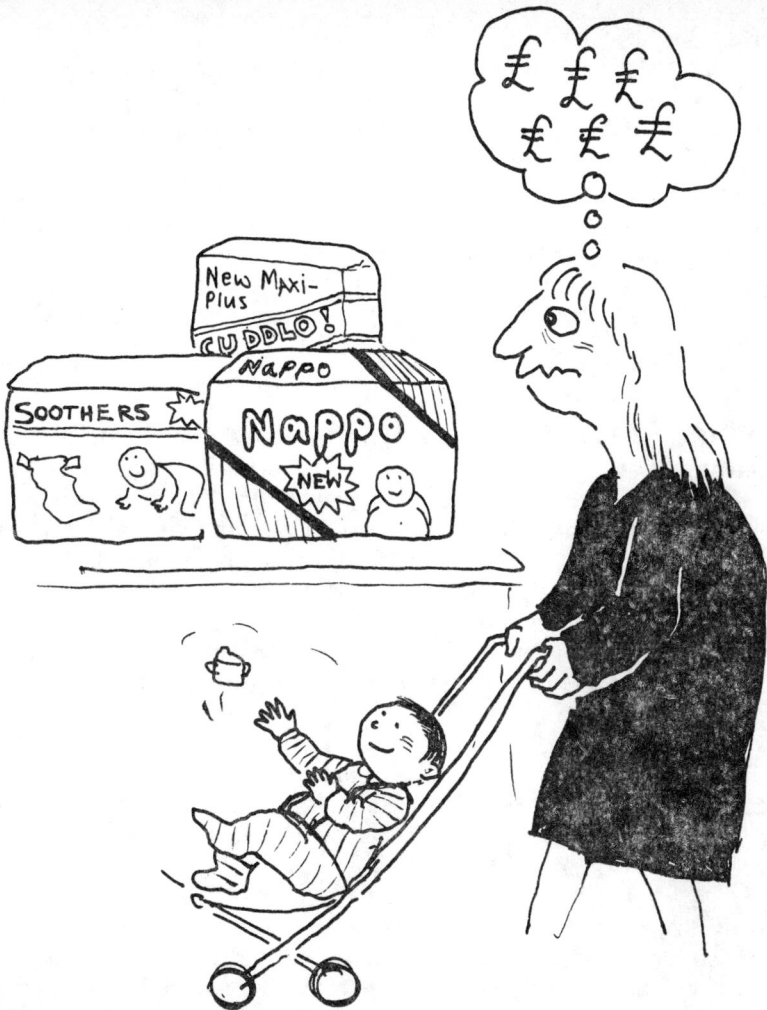

They may strain and cry, going quite purple in the face, and then relax when it is over. In time, as their digestive system matures, they will find the process a great deal easier. You can try giving a teaspoon or two of cooled mint tea but you will probably end up holding him against your shoulder and massaging his back as he squirms and strains. If this is a regular occurrence there is very little you can do other than wait it out.

WARNING SIGNS

Diarrhoea
This can very quickly become serious, particularly in a bottle-fed baby. You should get medical advice if stools change substantially, becoming looser than normal, perhaps watery-looking or full of mucous, and if they start to smell strange. In a fully breast-fed baby looseness without any other symptoms is rarely anything to worry about. *In all babies and young children speedy medical advice should be sought if looseness is accompanied by vomiting, loss of appetite and/or a temperature* (see Chapter 8 for more on this).

Greenish stools
These should not last more than four or five days after birth, or until milk feeding is well established (less with bottle-fed babies). If your baby's stools are not a pretty uniform yellow by the fifth day it could be a sign that breast-feeding is not well established and you might like to get advice from a midwife or breastfeeding councillor (see p. 101). If greenish stools return at a later stage (before you introduce other foods which could affect the colour), especially if your baby is not gaining weight well, you should mention this to a doctor or health visitor as it may be a sign that the baby is not getting enough to eat.

Blood spots
In the first few days of life these are common in girl babies. They are a response to the withdrawal of their mother's hormones after the birth. Any blood in the nappy at any other time should be reported to your doctor.

Constipation
This is most unlikely in a breast-fed baby but it can occur in bottle-fed babies and babies and children on mixed food. The major test of whether a baby is constipated is whether or not the stools are hard. If they are soft and easily passed then you should not worry even if they are a little irregular. Hard stools which cause the child distress need attention. Your health visitor or doctor can give you advice about a bottle-fed baby. You may need to change to a different formula.

With a baby or child on mixed food you will probably be able to sort the problem out yourself by increasing the amount of fruit and vegetable and, in particular, liquid in the diet. Don't give bran to a young child as it is very abrasive. Prunes or prune juice are a more gentle, natural laxative and usually very effective. If this doesn't work talk to your doctor. A child who has pain passing stools should see a doctor. Whatever is causing the pain needs attention because otherwise the child may try to avoid passing stools and this in turn will lead to constipation and greater pain.

Infrequent urination

This could be serious, particularly in a young baby. In the early months a baby should pass urine at least every two hours. If after four hours the nappy is still dry you should contact your doctor or health visitor as this may be evidence of an obstruction. If a baby is not wetting nappies frequently, or a child's urine is scanty and dark coloured they may be getting insufficient liquid to drink.

In a *breast-fed baby* who is gaining weight well, additional liquid is rarely necessary, so check that your baby is not over-wrapped (see p. 184) or feverish (see p. 203). If the weather is unusually hot or you have just turned on the central heating, you may need to feed more frequently or give a little additional liquid (very dilute fruit juice or boiled, cooled water) in a bottle. If her weight gain is also low you may need to discuss the whole issue of feeding with your doctor or health visitor. If none of these things apply and the urine is dark or has a funny smell there may be an infection for which you need medical advice.

If you are *bottle feeding* you should start by ensuring that you are mixing the feeds correctly. Adding extra formula to the water can cause dehydration. If you are sure that you are mixing the feeds correctly but the baby is still wetting infrequently try increasing the amount of water added to a feed (the baby will drink more but get the same amount of food). Check also that the baby is not overwrapped (see p. 184) or feverish (see p. 203). If wetting is still infrequent and the urine smells strange, ask the doctor to check for a urinary infection.

Older children may forget to drink as much as they need. If the urine is very dark in colour and your child's skin seems unusually sallow or dull and dry with shadows under the eyes, try to increase the amount he drinks during the day. Reluctant drinkers may like to use a straw or enjoy the addition of fizzy mineral water to fruit juice.

Frequent urination

In a young child who already has bladder control, frequent peeing and 'accidents' can simply be a response to cold weather. However, it can also be evidence of a mild urinary infection. The solution is *not* to reduce liquid intake but to increase it as much as you can and keep the child warm. This way, if there is some mild urinary infection you stand a good chance of flushing it out. If the frequency was caused by cold you will deal with that too. You will need loads of spare dry clothes to cope with this as the one thing you want to avoid is cold, wet knickers.

Painful peeing

This is usually a sign of infection. If it is accompanied by a temperature you need immediate medical advice. With or without a temperature you need to get as much liquid as possible into your child to flush the urine through. If your child has nappy rash or a vaginal infection (see p. 136) the acidity of the urine on the sore skin may be causing the pain. Again get her to drink as much as possible to reduce acidity while you deal with the rash (see below). If there is no rash and extra liquid doesn't ease the problem in a matter of hours, you should get medical advice.

Solids in – solids out

Once you introduce solids to a baby's diet the frequency of stools will usually settle at about once a day and it can be pretty predictable: just after breakfast or just after lunch. The colour and smell will change too. Any highly coloured food will show up, otherwise it will probably change to a pretty uniform brown. Observation will tell you what she is too young to digest: it will come out whole. A little undigested food will do no harm as long as she is getting enough food that she can digest easily (see Chapter 5).

Nappy changing can become quite a production as the baby's system adjusts to the new diet. The removal of a yellow stained nappy is a breeze compared to the full-scale strip which is often required now. Shit which is ejected at high speed can find its way right down into a baby's socks and halfway up her back: a good reason for avoiding garments which have to be removed over the head!

As your child gets older these alarmingly erratic bowel movements will settle down. Stools will be passed about once a day and will eventually start to go straight down the toilet without any intervention from you.

THE NAPPY PHASE: WHAT DO BABIES NEED?

'It is 2 am in mid winter. My baby is sleepily feeding and I just want to snuggle back into bed. Do I really have to get up, strip him off (waking him up in the process) and change his nappy? If I just put him back to bed will he get terrible nappy rash or soak through and wake up frozen?'

I don't know if I was the only person in the world to have these doubts and anxieties. I do know that I felt much too embarrassed to ask anyone in case I was considered a total slob and a bad mother for even considering leaving my child to sleep in a soggy nappy. Since I do tend to veer a little on the slobbish side, the warm bed got the better of me. I can report that he did not get nappy rash and, when I ensured that his nappies were sufficiently reinforced, he did not wake up cold and wet either. In addition to this, he started to sleep through the night quite quickly once I stopped waking him up thoroughly by exposing his warm little body to the cold night air.

There are probably thousands of mothers who are needlessly waking their babies up all through the night to change their nappies simply because no one has told them that it is unnecessary. Hospitals still teach nappy changing as though it were a military exercise to be adhered to at all costs:

> *'We were taught to change our babies both before and after a feed. As a result the baby was either screaming with hunger and rage long before she got to the breast, or roused to full consciousness just before being put down to sleep – or both. It is hard to imagine where this advice came from as it accorded neither with the baby's requirements nor our own.'*

Current advice from the Royal College of Midwives is that:

> *'She [the mother] should be told that it is not essential to change her baby's nappy before he goes to the breast. (A baby should never be allowed to become distressed before the breast is offered.)'*

While this is better advice than it used to be it still doesn't deal with the thing that we all needed to know. What do our babies actually need? In time of course we all work it out for ourselves, but a little bit of useful information would have been a help!

Unless a baby has particularly sensitive skin, a wet nappy will do little harm as long as it is warm wet and not cold wet (though see 'Sore bottoms', p. 135). If the wet nappy is enclosed in warm clothing (or bedding) it is unlikely to be causing discomfort. If it leaks, and makes the clothes wet, your baby (and probably you too) will soon get cold and uncomfortable. On the other hand, a dirty nappy shouldn't be left for long because it may make the baby quite sore. Knowing this, you can confidently work out a way of managing that suits you.

Keeping your baby comfortable

Every baby is different. Some have insensitive hides which don't mind too much what you do as long as they are washed regularly. Others need loads of barrier cream to reinforce them against the acid in their urine and seem to go red if you leave a dirty nappy in contact with the skin for a minute. You will find out very quickly what kind of baby you have got, but to start with it is probably safest to be on the careful side.

Cleaning
Cleaning at every nappy change is the first line of defence against nappy rash. Warm water is the cheapest method, though baby lotion or baby wipes

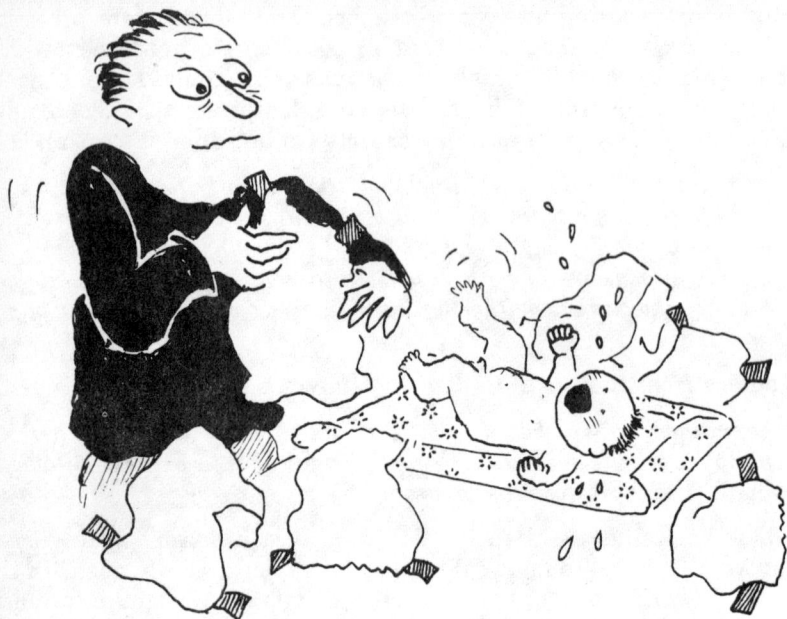

are useful for taking on trips. It's just as effective as anything else and probably more comfortable for a baby than icy cold lotions. If you keep nappy changing stuff in the bathroom (a board over the bath provides a changing platform) you can use cotton wool or a flannel for wet nappy changes and use the hand basin as a hip bath for more extensive cleaning. If you use a flannel make sure it is kept for the baby's bottom only and not used to wash her face. It should also be boiled regularly.

Waterproofing
This is definitely worthwhile in the early months, though you can experiment as the child gets older. Some don't seem to need it. Vaseline is as good as most things and most unlikely to cause an allergic reaction. Zinc and Castor Oil provides a thicker barrier for sensitive skins, though some children react to it. (Keep one hand cream-free if you use stick-on disposable nappies. Even a hint of cream on a sticker will render it sticky-less.)

Talcum powder
This should not be used at all. It serves no particular purpose and can easily be inhaled into the lungs. It also absorbs urine, keeping it in soggy rolls in the folds of the skin.

Nappy liners
These are not necessary if you use all-in-one disposables. Terry nappies rub if they do not have a liner. Disposable paper liners are cheap and effective but at night time a cotton 'one-way liner' is probably a better bet.

Double up
Use extra nappies or pads at night-time to ensure that your baby does not get wet through and cold. You can buy disposable nappy roll and cut off pieces to fit inside a terry or stick-on disposable nappy, or put a pad inside a one size larger disposable. As your child gets older, with more bladder control, you will probably find that a single nappy is enough. It is worth investing in good quality plastic pants. They last longer and work better.

Warm sleep suits
These provide better insulation if your baby regularly kicks the bedding off and gets cold.

Disposable nappies
These need to fit well around the legs to avoid leakage but should not be so tight that they rub. Different brands of disposables come in different sizes and shapes. Experiment until you find the one that suits your baby. Generally I have found that the more expensive, branded disposables are more absorbent than cheaper ones.

Terry nappies
These are just as absorbent (if not more so) than disposables and can be fitted to your baby's shape. If you do use them you need to be scrupulous about sterilising with fresh sterilant every day, or boiling them, or running them on the boil cycle of the washing machine (preferably drying them in fresh air), otherwise the nappies can harbour bacteria which cause nappy rash. Ecology-conscious parents may prefer terry nappies because they save on trees (however, on the minus side, washing them uses energy and sterilant pollutes the water supply – you can't win.) For more on hygiene, see p. 185–9.

SORE BOTTOMS

Redness in the nappy area, with or without little raised spots, should be treated as soon as it appears to stop it spreading.

Ammonia rash
The most common reason for nappy rash is ammonia, manufactured from urine by bacteria. You can usually smell the ammonia on the nappy. This problem is generally worse with terry nappies because ineffective sterilising fails to kill off the bacteria, which then multiply and

cause the rash. If a baby has very delicate skin you may get problems just from leaving a wet nappy in contact with the skin for a while.

To get rid of the rash you may need to change nappies more frequently for a few days. It will probably also help if you bath your baby in the morning and evening. If possible leave the nappy off for a while. Air seems to do wonders for nappy rash. When you replace the nappy make sure the baby's bottom is clean and dry and put plenty of barrier cream on to protect it.

Thrush
This may be the cause of a rash which simply won't go away. The thrush organism lives quite happily in the bowel most of the time and causes no trouble. Occasionally it multiplies and starts to cause an itchy rash around the vagina or anus, which becomes painfully red and angry. It can also affect the mouth (you can see the white patches), which may make feeding difficult. Antibiotics can cause an overgrowth of thrush or, since it is quite common for women to have thrush in their vaginas, it can be passed on at birth (or later if you are not careful about washing your hands). If your baby's rash does not seem to respond to ordinary precautions, go to a doctor. If thrush is not mentioned it may help to suggest it as it can be missed.

A cream containing an anti-fungal agent will be prescribed, which should work quickly. If it doesn't work go back to the doctor. There are many different kinds of anti-fungal cream and some seem to be more effective than others. It may also be that the thrush overgrowth in the bowel keeps recurring. If this is the case a liquid form of medication will be offered, which you can give on a spoon or in a dropper.

To prevent recurrences. If your baby is on solid food, it will help to give her live yoghurt to eat as it has anti-fungal properties. Try to keep nappies off when you can and change them frequently until the rash has completely disappeared. Constant enclosure in damp nappies encourages thrush to grow.

Vaginal soreness
This and irritation of the sensitive area around the vaginal opening can occur if a girl doesn't wipe herself properly after going to the toilet. This will be made worse if the knickers are made of nylon or some other synthetic substance. If she wears tights on top, the warm, damp environment makes a perfect breeding ground for infection.

If a child is prone to these infections she is better off wearing clothes which allow as much air circulation as possible. It is sensible to stick to cotton knickers. In cold weather, cotton leggings or loose trousers are less likely to cause problems than layers of synthetic materials. Regular baths with half a cup of vinegar in the water will sooth irritation and help to keep infection at bay. Avoid any other bath preparations and don't use soap to wash between her legs as it may cause further irritation.

If this simple treatment doesn't work the redness may be caused by thrush, in which case treatment similar to that described above may be necessary.

TOILET TRAINING

Getting your child to take responsibility for her bodily processes should not be a major difficulty. Most children are keen to grow up and see this as a step on the way. The object is to choose the time when they will find this achievement reasonably easy and unstressful. To a large extent this will depend on you being able to feel easy and unstressed about the process.

'I don't think I ever felt there was a particular age or time. I felt strongly that it was something I should not be too concerned about. When either of them had an accident after not wearing nappies I had a clear line that no negative response was called for. I think it worked well. Both my daughters went through the transition with little trouble and I found it completely stress-free.'

The second of these daughters came out of nappies at about two and a half, literally over one weekend. She was a highly articulate child who discussed the matter with her father on Friday and arrived at nursery the following Monday without nappies and completely confident of her ability to ask for the potty when she needed it. She had no accidents. In her case the combination of circumstances was ideal. Her father (her main caretaker) had made absolutely no issue about it and there was no external pressure. She was old enough to participate in the decision and had a high level of bladder control before she started using the potty. While these are conditions we all aim for, we don't always succeed so well:

'John had been out of nappies for a couple of weeks and we were doing pretty well. One day I arrived to pick him up from his childminder. He hadn't had a wee lately so I asked him to go – not wanting a sopping wet buggy on the way home. He refused point blank. I got irritated. He dug in his heels. I got more irritated. From that day he refused to pee in the potty at all and I was desperate. His minder suggested that I put the nappies back on, leave it a few weeks and start all over again. Next time round it went smoothly.'

Being calm and unfussed abut toilet training does help to make it relatively stress-free. Nevertheless, even neurotic parents usually get there in the end

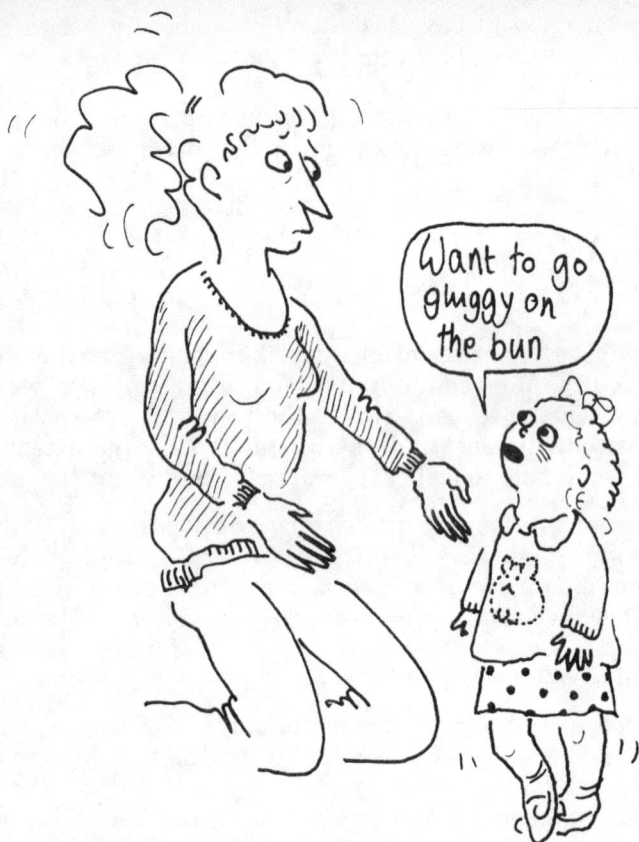

and not every peeing problem in an older child is traceable to bad early training. So if you simply cannot stop yourself from being annoyed the fourth time your child wets her knickers, do not assume that you are doing longterm damage! Personally, I was pretty hopeless at dealing with this stage but my children (so far) seemed to have sorted it all out in spite of me!

A word about words

As your child will be starting to talk at about the same time as she starts to use a potty, you will have to consider what you are going to call these bodily processes. Sometimes words just evolve and the family gets used to some bizarre and secret expression. Or maybe you believe in the playground approach and refer to piss and shit. Within your own family it doesn't matter at all what you call it, but it is worth keeping in mind that your child might need to use these words in another context and will depend on being understood.

'My friend and I were about to start our children together with a childminder. We had tended to refer to shit (as in "what a shitty nappy!") but we both decided to switch to wee and poo because that was what they were more likely to hear from other people.'

Getting started

Some parents have very strong feeling about the right time to start.

'My theory is that you leave them until the other side of two and a half even if they show signs of being interested before then or even if you want to get it done before a new baby comes. Both my children were dry and clean within two weeks with very rare accidents thereafter.'

'I think a child should be out of nappies by two and a half in the daytime and about three years at the night. It took me about eight weeks from starting – no problems.'

'So often I have seen children trained early use their pee or shit to provoke their parents and a child who was "quite good" at twenty months becomes still only "quite good" and not reliable at nearly three years old.'

Others find out by trial and error:

'I tried her when she was eighteen months but she kept crying. I tried again when she was two and she was very good. It took two weeks and she has never wet the bed and has been dry ever since. It was not a problem for her. She just did it.'

'The first time coincided with the warm weather and the obvious pleasure of seeing her running around without the vast encumbrance of terry nappies, and her pleasure of peeing directly onto the ground. We could talk about it and joke about it and she soon became aware that she could control it and always wanted me to know where she was peeing. She decided when she would wear a nappy. I think a child is "ready" when she can articulate in some fashion that she understands what is going on in her body. That is something that both the child and the parents can enjoy.'

In order to use a potty or toilet, a child needs to learn to control her bladder or bowel from the time it takes to feel the sensation and get to a potty. The object is to give the child control of this process and to see the attainment of control as a matter of pride. It is possible to force a child through this process by scolding if she fails and rewarding her if she succeeds, much as one would train a dog. However, if she sees the control of these things as coming from you and not from inside her, she will almost certainly lose control every time she is under stress and may well start using her ability to upset you as a way of controlling you too.

You can usually tell when a child has learned to recognise the happenings inside. He will stop and concentrate on the sensation and then resume whatever he was doing. Some children start to find their nappies uncomfortable when they are wet and dirty and ask to have them changed.

> *'My older boy is still in nappies (at twenty seven months). Although I would like him out I'm leaving it entirely up to him. He occasionally asks for the potty and he has started pulling at his clothes when he is wet. He loathes being wet or having poo stuck to his bottom.'*

Talk about it.

> *'I think children need to know that we adults pee and shit too. When I go to the loo myself I've always let them walk in. Also I talk about it; "Just a minute – I want a pee," or "Ooh! I'm hopping! Please be quick," then the children know that you have similar experiences.'*

Learning bladder control is not the same as learning bowel control. Bowel control ought to be easier because the sensations are stronger and the time between feeling the urge to poo and this actually happening is longer than the feeling of wanting to pee and the pee coming out. However, in practice the opposite may be true. Peeing is something that happens often. In a few days a child has many opportunities to practise controlling her pee and only one opportunity per day to do the same with her poo. She may also feel more anxious about the process of letting go of solid matter. This may be because the sensation of a full bowel comes quite a while before it actually appears and she is not quite sure when it will actually arrive. She probably also knows that you will be a lot less casual about a poo in the wrong place than you might be about the odd mis-timed pee.

> *'Sara learned very quickly to control her pee but I remember sitting around for hours waiting for a poo to come. She would feel something stirring and then hop off and on the potty for ages. I found it rather an anxious process because, though I didn't at all mind if she peed on the floor, the thought of shit on the sofa did not appeal.'*

Some children are so regular that bowel control is easy to attain:

> *'He was like clockwork. Every morning, as soon as he woke up, he would have a shit. When the time came to try a potty it was really easy – as long as I got up and helped him take his nappy off.'*

If a child spends time with older children the whole process is often much easier. This child was just two:

'With a couple of potties in the house, he learned in a matter of days. Self-taught I'd say, just encouraged, by me, but also by seeing the other children in the crèche and his elder half brother.'

Allow the potty to become a familiar object. Leave it around for a while before you expect your child to use it and explain in a matter-of-fact way what is is for. Your child may well want to experiment with it and become familiar with it before you take his nappies off and suggest he tries it.

If you have a garden toilet training can be very easy. It's just a matter of taking nappies off and leaving the child to run around with a bare bottom. That way the child can see the pee coming out and begin to relate the sensations from the inside to what is happening on the outside. Learning from what they see, it is a relatively short step to putting the pee in a potty. However, children are individuals. Some do not enjoy the sensation of nakedness and can get quite anxious about the possibility of pooing in an inappropriate place.

'Matthew got so wound up about the possibility of doing a poo that he refused to let us take his pants off even to go in the paddling pool. "Lappy," he would cry piteously, so we would put his nappy back on (pretty uncomfortable to paddle in). Once he felt confident about putting his poo in the right place this fear disappeared and he would happily run about naked and "water" the flowers in the garden.'

Toilet training in a fully carpeted flat may not be so easy as you are bound to feel anxious about accidents on the three-piece suite. In this case you may want to wait until you feel sure that your child is in charge of the process:

'I kept Tyrone in nappies until about three. He used to take them off himself to pee.'

Night time

Some children learn to control their bladder at night almost as soon as they have learned daytime control. They are so sensitised to the whole issue of peeing in the right place that they will wake with a dry nappy and call for a potty straight away. Jake simply refused to wear a nappy at all once he was dry by day:

'After a couple of wet beds and broken nights he has since been like me. Touch wood.'

Simply taking the nappies off will not always have this effect. If your child is not able to maintain bladder control all night you may simply have a wet bed to change every morning:

*'Rich refused to wear a nappy at night any more and we had wet beds
for the next five years.'*

If your child does wake dry and call for a potty it will help if you respond
immediately. For safety's sake you may want to keep the night nappy on for
a week or two but it is wise to be disciplined about responding promptly to
a call for a potty in the morning.

*'At the beginning he was dry every morning but we were a bit lazy
about responding to it and just left his nappies on. After a while he
went back to waking sopping wet every morning. Although he stopped
wearing daytime nappies at two and a half he is still wearing them
at night at four.'*

You will almost certainly get a few accidents even with the most easily
trained child. You will probably feel better about them if you prepare for
this possibility by putting a plastic sheet on the bed. You will also be glad
of an accessible change of night clothes and sheets in case your child wakes
up wet during the night.

Some children show no sign of night-time bladder control for some time:

*'At night he didn't stop wearing nappies until he was nearly four.
Friends advised "lifting" him when we went to bed. Result: screaming
child in a state about being disturbed. In the end we simply waited
until he had a couple of nights of being dry. Much happier scenario
for all and no bed-wetting since.'*

Lifting a child at night is a common, though not entirely logical, aid to
night-time dryness. Since the object is to accustom your child to going all
night without waking for a pee it is hard to see how lifting could do anything
except re-inforce regular night-time peeing. Obviously if your child refuses
nappies and still cannot either manage to wake up when he needs to pee, or
sleep through without peeing, lifting may be a labour-saving improvisation
to save the sheets. There is no other logical reason for doing it that I can
see.

Controlling evening drinking is not popular with child psychologists,
who argue that a child needs to learn to respond to her own bladder while
she is asleep and, by artificially cutting liquid intake, you are interfering
with a learning process. While I would certainly not advocate refusing all
drinks in the hours before bed I do think there is some sense in avoiding
overloading the bladder just before bedtime. I know that if I drink just before
bedtime I have to wake in the night to pee. Josie, now ten years old, found
that to be the solution for her:

*'I had to wear nappies at night till I was eight. I didn't like it so I
stopped drinking in the evenings and now I don't wear nappies any more
and hardly ever wet the bed.'*

External pressures

The things that conspire against a smooth transition are many.

Playgroups
If you know that your child will not be allowed to take up his playgroup place until he is 'dry' there will be inevitable pressure to 'succeed' at training. This anxiety is not surprising when child care of any kind is at such a premium and parents are desperate to get their children in to the few places that exist.

> 'At his playgroup they were supposed to be out of nappies and so I tried from his second birthday to get him ready. He came out of nappies (daytime) and by two and a half he was dry but he would still fill his pants as a regular occurrence (though not at playgroup). I over-reacted and used to get really angry with him. I know I dealt very badly with the whole situation. I just found it very hard not to be cross when he would go into another room and reappear with a bulky behind.'

In spite of this difficult start, this child quite quickly sorted things out and, now at school, has no further problems of this kind.

Parents' expectations
These set the tone for toilet training. If you are anxious it is hard not to pass your feelings on to your child. The mother quoted above found that her difficult first experience has damaged her own confidence and that could well affect the way she approaches toilet training with her young twins:

> 'I would hope that, if the weather permits, they can be in the garden. I intend to remove their nappies at two and see how it goes. I will try not to get angry with accidents and not to expect too much. I have to admit that I am dreading it.'

Friends and relations
They can either wittingly or unwittingly set up goals for you which have absolutely no relevance to your own child's readiness for toilet training:

> 'My mother-in-law must have had the only baby in the world that crapped to order! Quote: "I just held the potty there and. . . ." Not very helpful.'

Sometimes there is an age target which you feel you have to attain. Linda, with three children of her own and vast experience of many others, looks back with amusement on her own early ideas:

> 'I had a great idea that a child (baby) would be out of nappies by the age of one. With my first child I soon learned different.'

A new baby

You may rush into toilet-training your older child in order to ease the workload if a new baby is on the way. This can turn out to be far more stressful than simply changing an extra nappy. If you have to go with your child to the toilet each time she wants to pee (which you will need to do to start with), you may well find that a pee is required every time you sit down to feed the new baby. If you do not react calmly and quickly what started out as a real need could grow into a tactic for getting your attention.

Expense

The cost of nappies can also lead you to start training before your child is ready. If your training doesn't work you may find the need for extra clothes and the cost of washing is a higher price to pay than the extra nappies.

Travelling

This can be a real strain with a child who is just coming out of nappies:

'Going on the tube was a nightmare. I had his potty in a plastic bag and prayed that he wouldn't need it. Once, we had waited for ten minutes for a tube. As soon as it started he said he wanted a wee. I got off at the next stop and produced a potty but he said he didn't need it after all. It was hard to be calm in these circumstances.'

If you have to travel regularly with your child that may in itself be a good reason to start toilet-training fairly late, perhaps while you are on holiday. If your child starts to use a potty at a childminder's or nursery you can keep a nappy on for the journeys to start with but you will probably find that, within a short time, she simply won't pee in a nappy any more. If she allows you to put one on for the journey it will be more for your reassurance than hers. As soon as you do feel reasonably sure that she won't pee on your knee, trust her to take charge, but do take a spare set of clothing with you wherever you go so that accidents are not disasters.

'We were running for the train when he said "Mummy, I need a wee." Stupidly I didn't stop straight away but hoped he would hang on. Of course the poor little boy couldn't manage it. We missed the train and I had to buy a fresh set of clothes in a shop by the station.'

If you can be calm and sensitive to your child's needs, toilet training can be unstressful. If it takes your child six months longer than his friend you may feel a failure but you won't be. After all you do not, and cannot, control your child's bodily functions. This is not really a process of training but of watching your child mature and trying, as well as you are able, to be a help rather than a hindrance to something which is largely beyond your control.

'There is a lot of unnecessary hidden competition. From a very early

age the child becomes some kind of a trophy. The parents think they are doing things for the child when in fact they are doing it for themselves.'

COPING WITH PROBLEMS

It helps to decide first just when a child who is slow to achieve control has become 'a problem'. A child of three who has occasional accidents cannot really be described as having a problem unless a) there is a sudden regression, b) there is a distinct pattern, or c) you suspect that your child is refusing to cooperate rather than having difficulty in gaining control. Generally speaking boys are more likely than girls to run into trouble.

Achieving control

By four years old only 3 or 4 per cent of children have problems with bowel control. So it is reasonable to assume that if your child is still having serious difficulties at this age you could usefully start looking for help.

Starting school without proper bowel control is not necessarily a problem in itself but other children can certainly create one by teasing. Poor bladder control is a little more common at this age and may be looked upon with more forebearance by other children, but taunting is certainly not unknown.

According to the National Child Health and Education Survey 11 per cent of five-year-olds are regular bed-wetters and another 11 per cent do so occasionally. Night wetting is less likely to cause other social problems and so dealing with it may seem a lot less urgent. As long as your child is in nappies (larger incontinence pads are available on prescription when ordinary nappies get too small) night wetting need not become a problem for the entire household.

It will inevitably be more of an issue if you are coping with wet sheets every morning (and even more so if bed-wetting is causing disturbed nights.) If it is causing you irritation it is likely to become a source of stress for all concerned, in which case you would do well to seek advice. Otherwise there is no real rush, but do keep in mind the fact that bed-wetting can become a problem for an older child who would like to stay over at a friend's house but is embarrassed about her bed-wetting. So if your child is still bed-wetting at five, it might be in her interests to seek professional help.

Accidents and regression

Children who have achieved control may have accidents or even regress completely when under stress. Tension, fear or excitement may be the cause.

> 'John had been clean and dry day and night since he was two and a half. His occasional accidents were nearly always connected with some important event. Once when we were out shopping for birthday party food he soiled his pants. I was hopping mad at the time but realise now that it was the excitement that caused it.'

Some children seem to get so engrossed in playing that they 'forget' to go to the toilet, or leave it too long and end up making a last-minute dash.

> 'Ruth would be hopping from foot to foot but refused to go to the toilet and insisted that she didn't need to. Then she would have an 'accident' and I would get angry with her. Gradually I realised that I was taking responsibility for what should be her responsibility and I stopped nagging. Occasionally I would say very firmly "Ruth, you need to go to the toilet and if you have an accident I will be very annoyed with you." She would at first deny it and then, when I had dropped the subject would announce, as though I hadn't mentioned it at all, that she needed a wee. Once she felt in charge of things, the accidents were less frequent.'

You may need to help your child to take more control. For example, a step (or small plastic box) by the toilet may help her to use it unaided. If your only toilet is upstairs and the lights are off, she is most unlikely to make the journey unaided. Even if the lights are left on, a journey upstairs alone may seem alarming to a three-year-old. Providing a potty downstairs in an accessible place will encourage her to take charge of the situation on terms she can handle.

A child may start having accidents when she goes to visit a friend or starts playgroup or nursery for the first time. This may be partly a reaction to stress but it can also be very difficult to attract an adult's attention immediately when they are caring for twenty other children. Make sure that your child knows exactly where the toilet is and is wearing clothes that he can easily get off unaided. Most nurseries have a supply of spare clothes in case of accidents but, if you know that your child has a tendency to accidents when under stress, he may feel better knowing that a spare set of his own clothes is available for emergencies.

Greater stress, for example the birth of a sibling, parental separation or injury may cause more long-term problems with soiling, accidents or night wetting. Josie had been dry day and night for a year before her sister was born. She started wetting the bed and continued to do so for the next five years. In fact the birth of a sibling is a fairly common trigger for regression in bladder control, as Carole found:

> 'My oldest completely reverted when the new baby was born (he was three and a half) and actually used to pee on the floor in front of me when I was feeding. It didn't last long. I was able to deal calmly with the "more relaxed" attitude to the second baby in general.'

More serious problems

Wetting and soiling in children who 'ought' to be clean is often assumed to be an emotional problem. Other parents may well make remarks about children being 'pushed' too early or imply that the parents have 'caused' the problem by inappropriate handling. Of course this may be true but it is not the only reason for problems with toilet training. Children do not develop physically to order and problems can arise even in the most apparently 'laid back' households:

> 'I waited until the warm weather then started not putting nappies on them and taking them to the potty frequently. I had no problem with Anna who was two and a quarter but later when I did the same for Rich I was busier and perhaps less thorough with routines. Maybe he didn't feel ready (at two and three quarters). Rich went on being unreliable (peeing and shitting) until he was seven. I felt very bad about it and felt I hadn't established a calm enough climate. To resolve the problem I finally sought professional help.'

There are no obvious reasons for this mother's problems with her second child. It wasn't too early, he was not threatened or harrassed. He simply refused to do it. In fact, perhaps their only mistake was to wait as long as they did before seeking help, assuming that it was just a matter of time. In the event the problem was compounded by merciless teasing from other children which did not come to light for some time. The psychologist's view was that for many reasons, quite unconnected with toilet training, Rich had decided not to take responsibility for himself – he didn't want to grow up. After a short period of therapy he finally achieved control and learnt to take more responsibility for his life in other ways as well.

Rosie could have had similar problems, but being an exceptionally articulate child she was actually able to explain what she felt to her parents:

> 'I never attempted to toilet train her. I don't even remember now how old she was when she came out of nappies. She had worked out that you have to be "dry" to progress from the "baby" room to the "school" room at nursery. At one point, after she had control, she promised to

*stay dry if I still put her in a nappy so they wouldn't guess at nursery
and put her up to the other room – this aged two!'*

If a nappy represents safety and being looked after, it is not difficult to see
how a child who may be lacking confidence in other ways can use soiling
and wetting as a demand to be looked after – to be babied.

Medical problems

Urinary infection (see above) may cause loss of bladder control and constipation may be the cause of soiling. It is worth asking for a medical check
for persistent problems even if there are no other obvious symptoms.

GETTING HELP

Problems with toilet training are not uncommon. If time and patience are
not helping your child achieve control do not feel that you have failed. So
often with difficulties of this kind what you need is some support and advice
from people who are not emotionally involved with you or your child. It
would have been impossible for Rich's parents to have analysed and solved
their child's problem without help from outside the family. Once they had
that help a whole spiral of anxiety began to unwind. Your doctor will have
helped many other parents and, once she has established that there is
nothing clinically amiss, she may well refer you to an 'enuresis' clinic in the
area.

Chapter 7

CARE SHARING

James James
Morrison Morrison
Weatherby George Dupree
Took great
Care of his Mother
Though he was only three.
James James said to his mother,
'Mother,' he said, said he;
'You must never go down to the end of the town, if
you don't go down with me.'
(A. A. Milne, When We Were Very Young)

LOVING, BONDING AND DROWNING

As a generation of parents we are bombarded with totally conflicting information about our relationship with our children. On the one hand women are told that they should exclusively breastfeed their babies for as long as possible and made to feel guilty about leaving them with anyone else. On the other hand they are expected to be career women, ready to leave their children and return to fulltime work as soon as possible.

Caught between these two different roles, women often find that they get insufficient support for either function. Partners expect them to be housekeeper, mother and lover rolled into one and very often wage earner on top. Employers expect them to be immediately ready to return to work without any concessions to the demands of being a parent. Health and social service personnel expect them to be ever available carers, ready to turn up to three-hour appointments in the middle of the day. Frequently it feels as though the only real support comes from other mothers under much the same degree of pressure as themselves.

Men also face complicated contradictions. They may intend to take a real share in child care yet often the lack of provision for parental leave at work means that, after the first few days, they have little contact with their babies. They may also find that the only effective means of soothing their baby is not available to them because their partner is exclusively breastfeeding. Given the lack of social pressure on them to persist in finding ways of involving themselves, they too often find it easier to opt out altogether rather than confront their own helplessness. As Sheila Kitzinger observes in her book, *The Crying Baby*:

> *'Many fathers accept their share of baby-care in the first weeks but, on realising that the woman can do everything better, they give up. They retire behind a newspaper or go off for a drink and leave the woman to get on with it.'*

The more a mother is left alone with her new baby the more intense the bond may become, and the more exclusive the relationship the harder it may be to stand back and allow someone else to take over. Even when she is under extreme pressure she may find herself excluding her partner from the care of their child by accentuating his feelings of incompetence rather than providing the space in which he can develop his own relationship – and make his own mistakes. After all, as one father was quoted saying in *The Crying Baby*:

> *'When I began looking after my son I came crashing up every day against the limits of my masculine upbringing. Nothing in my life experience, nothing I had observed in other men or my father prepared me for doing this job.'*

Vince looked after his daughter for half the time right from the start. He remembers:

> *'The key moment was when I went to pick them up from the hospital. I started changing her nappy and putting on her babygro. If Sheila had interfered it would have been disastrous but she didn't. We both knew it was important.'*

Sharing care with a partner or member of your family is pretty easy compared to giving your child over to someone you hardly know. Of course our children need the security of our love and we need to be sure that the people we leave them with will really *care* about them. However, we can get so wrapped up with our babies that we cannot entertain the thought of someone else helping to look after them. This mother genuinely believed that:

> *'It would be impossible to leave her with anyone else because I am the only person who really knows her well enough to judge when she needs to sleep. She may have several half-hour naps during the day. If she doesn't get them, she will be tired and difficult and I don't want that to happen.'*

An experienced childcare worker should have no difficulty in working out when a baby is tired and reacting accordingly. This mother was under no financial pressure to return to work and deeply resented what she saw as pressure from other parents to do so. Perhaps she was afraid to accept that someone else could care for her baby because that would mean accepting that she do something else. Her anxiety was caused by her own fear of separation, not her child's. We fear losing our children because we love them. Maybe we are also remembering our own fear of being left when we were children. Yet we know, from other experiences, that we can love people without being glued to them twenty-four hours a day. One of the most comforting things a friend ever said to me at this time was:

> 'Having a baby is like having a love affair. You hate to part in the
> morning but you do it knowing that you will come back together
> again still loving one another but refreshed from being apart.'

With very young babies the sense of loss is compounded by anxiety for their welfare – after all they cannot tell you if they are not happy. They are powerless without your presence. However, the wrench will be there at whatever age you leave them, even if you have longed for a break and are delighted to have time to yourself at last. Mothers leaving their five-year-old children at school for the first time often talk about the tears they shed as the door closes. The difference is that, at five, society is not only supporting this separation, it is backing up that support with the full force of the law.

At a younger age, at least in Anglo-American societies, separation has only recently begun to be socially sanctioned. In spite of the enormous changes in the way women live and work now, compared to their mothers' generation, leaving a young baby in someone else's hands is a break with convention. Mothers from cultures in which child care is more of a communal activity are under less pressure in this respect. A Carribbean mother said:

> 'My mother worked, my grandmother worked, why shouldn't I go out
> to work too?'

Her feelings were backed up by a young woman I spoke to who had been brought up in Sweden:

> 'Everyone's mothers worked. That was just the way life was. It wouldn't
> occur to me to feel guilty about going out to work. It's normal.'

MORE THAN MOTHER

Women in the UK, perhaps more than anywhere else in the world, have been brainwashed with the theory of maternal deprivation. It is an idea developed by pyschiatrist John Bowlby, who worked with children separated for long periods of time during the war. His work soon provided the basis for World Health Organisation documents about the care of children, and the evidence for the closure of many wartime day nurseries.

Bowlby believed that children separated from their mothers, even for a short period of time, could be permanently damaged emotionally. This was pretty strong stuff and the ideal weapon for getting most war mothers out of the work force and back into the kitchen.

While he was right about a baby's need for consistent, loving care and contact, there is nothing to support his theory that a baby would suffer if she was left for short periods of time with another responsible, caring adult. Indeed, according to anthropologist Margaret Mead, the idea that primitive societies allow for a continuous, unbroken, and therefore 'natural' mother-child bond until the child is two is simply not borne out in practice:

'Under primitive conditions there are two situations which require a break in the continuity of mother-child care: a) the need of the other children for care, and b) the demands on the mother for food gathering, horticultural and other contributions to the food supply of the family group.' (quoted in Caroline New and Miriam David, *For The Children's Sake*, Pelican, 1985)

Mead maintained that it is only in a society which practises contraception, and in which most food production takes place outside the home, that such total togetherness is feasible. In other words, we have invented an idea of what is 'natural' which would be impossible to achieve in a non-industrialised society. It is in fact extremely unusual for a human baby to have only one caretaker and almost unheard of for this exclusivity to last beyond the early months when a baby is dependent on frequent breastfeeding. According to research quoted in *The Care of Young Children*, a booklet by Professor Barbara Tizard of the Thomas Coram Research Unit:

'Out of 186 contemporary, non-industrial societies there were only five where the child was almost exclusively looked after by the mother.'

This does not mean that a single exclusive bond is wrong but it does throw doubt on the assumption that, because it is what *we* do, it must be right. There is no absolutely right way. Children are brought up to fit into a particular society and they are expected to adapt to the social norms of that society. In Anglo-American societies individuality is prized and competitiveness is fostered. Our form of child-rearing is adapted to that form of social organisation. In a country which prizes cooperation above competition, this form of social organisation would be counterproductive.

When different sorts of social organisation get mixed up children may well get confused. For example, most African societies are far more cooperatively organised. Family members take a lot more responsibility for the common care of children and they are loved, played with and disciplined by a larger group of people than is usual in, for example, Anglo-American communities. African and Caribbean parents in the UK may be shocked and disappointed when they discover that other adults do not automatically participate in the care of their children.

Differences are apparent even between European cultures. A friend of mine moved to Italy shortly before having her child and was quite amazed by the childcare conditions that Italian women considered to be not only quite normal but admirable:

> 'I could have got a place in a day nursery for her but there seemed to be so many other children that I didn't want to do it. The Italian mothers think nothing of it, they are quite happy to leave their children with twenty others and go off to work.'

Italian day care is widely considered to be a model for child care in Europe. Nursery design is very advanced, there is much lively discussion about what children can and should learn in the first three years of life, and a real sense of the importance of child care. However, once children start to walk, they do not insist on such a high ratio of adults to children as we normally do in the UK. An Italian nursery nurse explained their philosophy:

> 'We are not trying to provide substitute mothering. We do not want to imitate the mother-child relationship. We feel we should encourage relationships between the children, more than between adults and children.'

When we, as parents, think about what we want for our children we are thinking mainly about what we had as children and assuming that it must be best. To step outside the territory of our own personal experience is to step into the unknown and it makes us feel anxious. Will our children cope? Are we imposing impossible strains on them? It might help us get perspective on our decisions to know that French mothers often send their children to nursery school at two and a half years old in groups of twenty or more while Swedish three year olds usually remain in groups of seven children to an adult until they start school when they are seven. In the UK we may keep our children at home until they are nearly five and then throw them in at the deep end with a group of thirty. Who can claim to be right?

With so little certainty how do we make decisions for ourselves and our children? It may help if we can start to establish just where our children's needs end and our own needs begin.

WHAT DO WE NEED?

Time for ourselves

We all need time for ourselves. Time to renegotiate relationships with our partners, to get perspective on our lives, to engage with the outside world

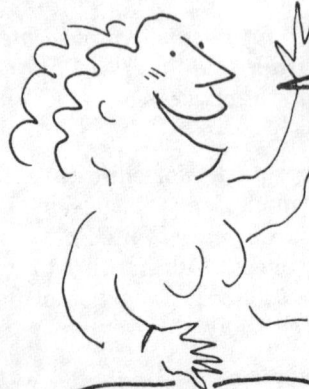

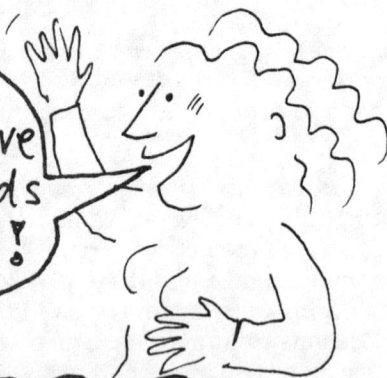

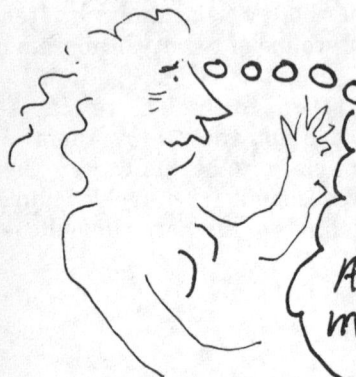

and, increasingly, time to earn a living too. The time we need for ourselves requires that we hand over control of our children to someone else. It may just mean leaving a partner or friend in charge for brief periods during evenings and weekends. It may mean a genuine division of child care between parents. It may mean handing over our children to the care of another person, or people, for extended periods while we work.

Even when our own needs overwhelm us and we desperately need some space, we may find it hard to ask for it. Isabella remembers:

'I was very depressed for a long time when Paulo was little and that didn't help with our relationship. I was sort of crippled emotionally. I could manage the practical things but it was as though my heart was somewhere else. It was like my soul being imprisoned and incapable of real warmth.'

Isabella did not attempt to find child care until Paulo was two. She feels now that she left it too late.

'It wasn't hard at all to leave him though he cried a lot in the beginning . . . I was dying to have time on my own but I felt guilty because I was so relieved.'

Susan felt able to leave her child in a nursery at twelve months. She now thinks, in retrospect, that it could have been sooner:

'I felt relieved since it was such a wonderful place and I had turned into a "non person", having taken a year off work and stayed home because, at thirty-nine, I thought it would be best all round. Now I think he would have benefited from being there at six months and so, I now see, would I.'

Jan had very little access to child care, other than informal swops with other mothers, until her children started school:

'The best things have been that I have spent a lot of time with the children up to them starting school and seen a lot of that development (my husband has missed that, being at work, and he regrets the loss). The worst is that I have been through a total crisis of confidence because I was out of fulltime work for eight or nine years.'

For most women in the UK, carving out time away from the children is a major problem. We have the lowest level of childcare provision of any country in the Common Market other than Ireland. Nursery schools are not universally available and, when they are, the standard 2½-hour session barely gives us enough time to get there and back again. As a result, British mothers of young children are more likely than most to be working very short hours for very low pay, in jobs which are often well below our level of skill.

Partners do little to help. Jake chose to stay home while his wife went to work because she earned considerably more than he did. At first he did all the domestic work and the child care and did not expect to do any of his own work. As the children got older he arranged alternative child care for several hours a day. However, he says:

'I would find that, at the weekends, she would just announce that she was going shopping, and walk out the door. I had been looking after the children all week without a break and had no free time to myself. In the end we had a real row, and then started trying to renegotiate. Now she takes overall responsibility on Saturdays and I take overall responsibility on Sundays. We often do things together but at least I know that, if I want to just go out on Saturday afternoon, I don't have to ask permission.'

Since women more often than men do the main share of caring it is they who are more likely to find themselves in this position. According to government statistics published in 1989 (Social Trends 1989, HMSO), women employed part-time have considerably less leisure time than men employed full-time. Women employed full-time with husbands who are also employed have least leisure time of all – three-quarters of them do most of the housework on top of their paid work. One major way for women (whether they work or not) to achieve more time for themselves is to insist on a more equal division of domestic labour.

Alternatively we can find other ways of living together. Marcia's family are from the Carribbean. She has never lived with the father of her child but nor has she been alone:

'I've had immense support from my parents. Ebony has always seen them regularly and they have always been around – part of the network of people who love me and care for me. They bring a track record of their own security about being parents.'

Marcia would find it very hard to manage her stressful, full time job without this loving support.

Time with our kids

Rapidly changing attitudes to working women and a greater than ever economic need for women to stay in work when they have children means that many of us are facing a new problem. We are leaving our children sooner and for longer than we feel comfortable with.

If we are returning to work we need *a supportive work environment* if we are to feel sure that we can balance our own needs, the needs of the job, and the needs of our children. This supportive atmosphere is slow to grow:

*'My second child was struggling for life and I had to go back to work
for the money. I asked for extra paid leave in what I consider unusual
circumstances. The request was denied. I also asked for permission to
work a 3–4 hour day until the situation resolved itself. The request was
denied.'*

It is hard to imagine anything less supportive than this, reported in the
Maternity Alliance book *The Inside Story* (see the bibliography on p. 216).
Yet many new parents have to put up with reactions ranging from hostility
to blank incomprehension. Employers are often unwilling to adapt to our
needs and colleagues may even complain about time taken off to care for
sick children. The effort of adapting a child-led schedule to a work-led one
can be emotionally exhausting. Researchers worry about women's lack of
motivation and failure to put themselves forward for top jobs. Most of us are
exhausted by the effort of staying in one place. We don't have time to think
about the next step. This need not be so. The workplace can adapt to the
needs of a society in which both parents work. (See p. 179 for more about
changing working conditions).

For Haley, the combination of stress and guilt outweighed the rewards.

*'I left my son with a childminder at ten months. I felt very upset and
guilty though I don't think it bothered him. I swore that if I ever had
another child I wouldn't go out to work. You miss all their growing
up and their funny little ways.'*

Haley decided to take up childminding herself so that she could stay at
home. Many women simply stop outside work for a period of months or years
in order to look after their children themselves. While this option may sound
attractive (to those with the economic security to do it), it is not necessarily
the complete solution. Most women in the UK do want to go back to work
at some point and a complete break can make it very difficult. Jan, who was
quoted earlier, found that her self-confidence completely collapsed when her
youngest child started school. Faced with the thought of returning to her
own work she found herself sucked into a depression which was only resolved
by a course of psychotherapy.

Jan was lucky – as a self-employed designer she had only to build up
her own self-confidence in order to make the breakthrough. Most of us have
to convince our prospective employers that a few years at home has not
addled our brains. If we don't have confidence in our own abilities it will be
hard to inspire confidence in others. On committees where I have had to
scrutinise job applications I have been amazed at how clearly the low self-
esteem of many women shows through their applications. Men who have
taken time out to care for children may have the additional problem of
employers who feel deeply suspicious about the motivation of a man who
makes this decision.

Support

Partners need to be particularly aware and supportive at the time we return
to work. Whether it is after a few weeks or a few years, the change from the
total absorption in child care to the outside world of work is usually hard.
Of course many of us welcome it but few with such equanimity as Trish,
who said:

> 'On my first day back I felt released. It was wonderful and I came home
> refreshed. I never had any hesitation about leaving my children in the
> care of others. I am not too good with babies. I prefer them as they get
> older so I always assumed that, provided the alternative care was
> good, they would be doing better than they could with me.'

If you have been at home for some time, finding the confidence to reorganise
your life may not be easy. However, there are now many more courses aimed
specifically at women returners (the major employment agencies often run
their own and the Manpower Services Commission can provide information
on skill training). These courses are aimed as much at confidence building
as anything else. More employers (particularly in the finance sector) now
arrange 'work breaks', which allow parents to keep in touch with their
workplace while at home with children and give them priority for jobs at
their own skill level when the time comes to return.

WHAT DO CHILDREN NEED?

Attachment

If you leave a baby of eight months alone with a complete stranger she will
almost certainly be upset. A nursery nurse observed:

> 'It used to be much easier settling the babies when their mothers were
> going back to work after three or four months. Now they are getting
> longer maternity leave and bringing them at seven or eight months
> and it takes longer for them to get used to us and settle down.'

Somewhere between six and eight months, a baby starts to become aware
that her principle caretakers are not actually attached to her – she can lose
them. This realisation is frightening. Some distress at being left alone with
a stranger is likely to persist until the child is three and can continue in
some form or another for a great deal longer. This is probably a basic safety
mechanism which protects the child from getting lost and keeps her within
safe range of people she knows and trusts.

However, just because a child is upset by being left with someone she

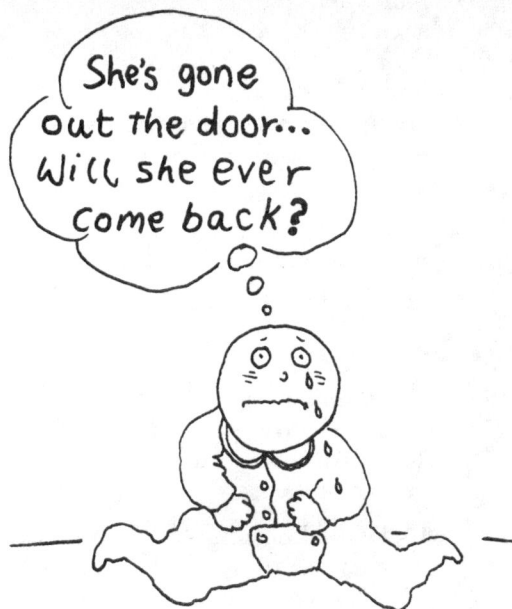

does not know, there is no reason to avoid leaving her with someone she does know. In fact it probably helps for a child to get to know several adults early on because that is the best protection against having to be left with a stranger. All the parents I have spoken to who have made alternative child-care arrangements believe that it is for the child's benefit as well as their own. One commented:

'I wish we had adult friends they were really close to – a potential second family, in case something happened to us.'

The issue is not whether a child should spend time with other people but just how best to help our children make additional, safe relationships.

Secondary attachments

Mot children start off by getting very attached to their mother, a few fix primarily on their father or another relation who cares for them, and some seem to be equally attached to both parents. However, they are also forming secondary attachments with anyone who regularly appears in their lives.

When their most important person leaves they will be distressed, but as long as they are left with someone to whom they are also attached, the distress will be short-lived. A nursery worker commented:

'Matthew, at eighteen months, always raised the roof when his mother

*left him. He would cling on to her and cry piteously. She would have
to quite literally unwind herself from him. It was very hard for her but
we reassured her that, within minutes of her leaving, he would be
busy and happy. The message was quite clear: he didn't like her to
leave but, if he failed to prevent her from leaving he was perfectly
content to get on with something else. Far from being damaged by it,
he was slowly learning that other adults could be trusted. There was
life outside mother.'*

Once attachments are formed with other people they offset the fear of being
left. Children may form a clear hierarchy of attachments: mother first, followed by father and then siblings or close relations, followed by non-family
members, each degree of closeness being more comforting than the last:

*'Two-year-old Julia would throw a wobbly if she was left alone with
me at the end of the day. She would accept my care only if her big
brother was there too. He patiently accepted the situation and agreed
to act Daddy for the hour until they were all picked up.'*

A child who is being breastfed will almost inevitably be more closely attached
to his mother and may be reluctant to stay with his father. A father who
does not understand the process of attachment and is not prepared to take a
longterm view of parenting may find this distressing, interpret it as personal
rejection and, as a result, withdraw from close contact leaving more and
more child care to the mother. Berni found himself cutting off from the two
younger children during the first year and concentrating on the older ones.
Sandra was aware of the growing distance and, he noticed:

*'She manipulated the situation a bit with the middle one and I've
noticed her doing it again with the baby. Just as they get to tottering
stage she starts to disappear and leave me alone with them. I suppose
she is deliberately trying to foster closer contact as she starts to wean
her.'*

For Berni the slight distance during the baby stage has not been a problem.
He is very committed to fatherhood and was perfectly content to wait it out
until the babies became small children and started to return his affection.

Encouraging attachment

When you introduce your child to a new carer you will have to give them
time to get to know each other. If you make the introduction before six
months and she sees him regularly, she will probably just absorb that new
person into her life. When she starts to be concerned about separation she
will already consider her new carer one of the important adults in her life
and you will probably experience little difficulty in leaving her.

'Ruth started with her minder at four months. I worried about her, she

*didn't worry about me. Since then her minder's family has become
her second home. She is fortunate to have two homes and a second set
of brothers and sisters. I can really think of nothing about the
arrangement that has not been a plus for her.'*

Ruth's minder has this advice to other mothers going back to work:

*'Start looking as soon as the baby is born. If it is going to a childminder
a relationship can be beginning even if it is only one afternoon a week,
or a few hours.'*

Mary, a General Practitioner with three children, found that:

*'Baby three stayed with me for eight months. He reacted very badly to
the childminder. I feel it was my fault. I left it too late.'*

For those over six months it is important to introduce the new situation
gradually if you can. It will certainly be easier for you to go back to work
knowing that your child is happy rather than having to shut the door on a
howling, distressed child. Rosanne was ten months:

*'It took a while to get arrangements settled but it is now really good.
We did it gradually after a completely wrong first few attempts when
they were alone for some hours with no preparation. So for a few weeks
I paid Vivien to be here when I was. It seemed silly at the time – two
grown women caring for a little baby – but it worked.'*

If money is going to be very tight during your maternity leave it may be
worthwhile seeing if you can return part-time for the first few weeks (going
back a little earlier if necessary) just so that you can get things going
gradually. If you are lucky your carer will be happy for you to visit regularly
before you start work:

*'We had two babies who visited the crêche regularly with their mothers.
By the time they were a few months old they were quite clearly
enjoying their visits. Both of them started to come alone, regularly,
when they were a little over nine months. They took to it with
enthusiasm.'*

Consistent care

Changing carers is certainly not ideal but it can rarely be avoided altogether.
Few children who are being cared for by people outside the family are
fortunate enough to have one set of carers or one place to get used to.
Childminders stop minding, nannies leave and very few children get into
nurseries before the age of two. The important thing is to be aware that
your child will react to a change. Each change needs to be approached with
as much care as the first one, as this mother discovered.

'Alan was going to school at 9.30 and then staying to playcentre until 5.30. It was the same length day as his nursery had been but after school he would be impossible, kicking me, having tantrums. I was in tatters and finally went to see his teacher in despair and burst into tears.'

The teacher suggested that the problem lay in the enormous change between the day nursery with an adult to every five children, and a school with one or two adults to thirty children. Had Alan attended a school nursery, with a lower level of adult involvement, he would probably have been able to make the transition more easily. He would have started learning how to relate to his peers directly, without always having an adult to intervene. As it was he took out his anger and misery on his mother.

Jerome went through four individual carers and three different groups in his first three years. The changes were well spaced out and these nannies have returned since to babysit in the evenings. He sees many of the children whom he met in his first group and he seems to have taken it all in his stride. His mother is the most important person in his life and, as long as she has time to spend with him in the evenings and weekends, he seems to cope. His mother says:

'Getting them used to a new nanny is hell, but once settled the baby is happy. The older one grumbles about me going off to work but soon settles and is sociable and articulate and has an independence which he wouldn't have if he had only been with me.'

However, two year old Paul could not cope with continually being shunted from pillar to post:

'I had been at work for twelve years when I had Paul. I went back when he was 7 months and he just didn't settle with the first minder so I moved him. The second one's child got ill so I had to move him again. The third gave up and went to work herself and by the fourth, he just wasn't settling at all so I gave up work.'

Paul's mother stayed at home for a year and then returned part-time when she judged that her son felt more secure.

Leaving work may well not be an option for you, so it is important to handle changes in caretaker sensitively. Even if you are also under pressure at work, try to make time to be with your child, talk about the person who has been lost, explain where they have gone to and, if possible, arrange occasional visits so that your child does not feel abandoned.

Quality time

Children need special people in their lives. They need to know that they come top of somebody's list. There is no reason why they should not spend a big dollop of time each day with someone who loves them even if their parents go out to work. In fact, parents who go out to work may give their children more 'quality time' because they are not endlessly devising ways of getting them out of the way, distracting them, and shushing them in order to carve out some space for themselves.

Berni and Sandra both have jobs which take them away from home on occasion and involve evening meetings. However, they consider parenting to be a joint project and make sure that it is given time. Says Berni:

'I don't do anything between 5 pm and 7 pm unless it is absolutely necessary. That time is for the children. They are my first priority. I enjoy that and wouldn't miss it for the world. It is what life is about. I do come under pressure to stay on sometimes but meetings at 6 pm are in my opinion just a way of spending time before going to the pub. They are an excuse to avoid domestic responsibility.'

Sharing responsibility for the evenings provides a great deal more flexibility for parents, as well as much more organisation. Says Sandra:

'We compare diaries monthly and update them weekly. If I have something big coming up which will take me away from home I make sure it is in his diary well in advance. We try to make sure that we are both here at teatime and then, if we have evening meetings, we get a babysitter but we always put the children to bed before we go out. In fact in six years they have only once been put to bed by anyone else.'

These parents are lucky to live within half an hour's driving distance of work. The problems are much greater if one or both parents commute.

Single parents have to find the energy to provide special times by themselves, though sometimes another adult will welcome the opportunity to become a special friend and spend a regular evening with a child. If time during the day is at a premium and you are not in a position to negotiate time off you might want to consider sleeping with your child. Those early morning moments of waking together can be worth a great deal in establishing a real loving closeness. It is the feeling of being special, being listened to, being the focus of attention that is so important. (See 'Changing work', pp. 179–81, for ideas on how to change your working hours.)

Time without us

The very intensity of the parent-child relationship can create pressures which children may well be glad to be free of for a while.

'My children always feel a little cheated when their favourite babysitter comes, if I don't leave home soon enough for them to spend time alone with her.'

This doesn't mean that they love us any the less, merely that they need space for themselves just as we do. This is just as true for the child in a large family as for the lone child. Barbara Tizard explains:

'Sibling [brother and sister] interactions are more highly charged emotionally than peer relationships, with more aggressive behaviour, but also more affectionate, helping, cooperative behaviour. Sibling roles are much less equal than peer roles, and for this reason there is an obvious advantage to children in having relationships with peers as well as siblings.'

It should not be difficult for us to identify with our children's need to be free of us. We would find life pretty limited if we were forced to spend all our time with one or two other people (even if we loved them dearly).

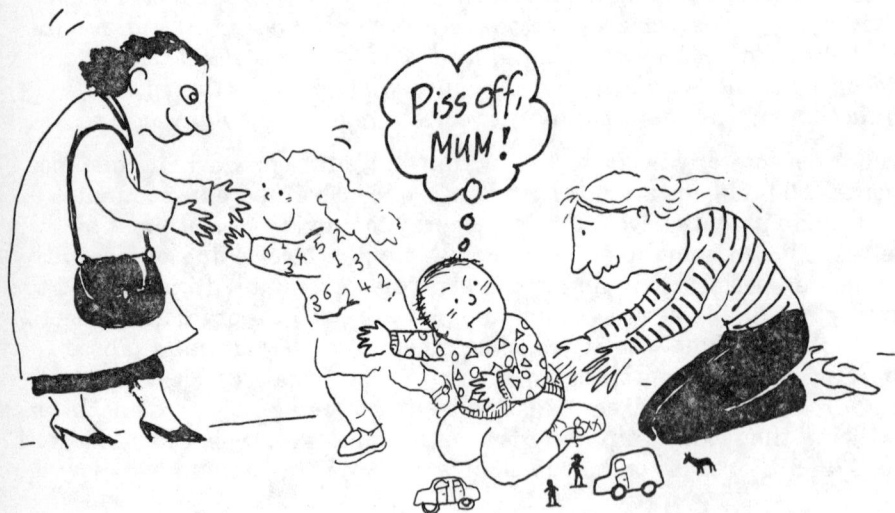

'I have watched withdrawn, frightened children, who clutched their mother's skirts when they first came to the crèche, gradually opening up and starting to join in. It is not just their behaviour which changed. They seemed to look different too: more confident, happier, taller!'

SWOPS, FRIENDS AND SHORT-TERM CARE

Even if you are not leaving your child to go out to work it is important to deal with separation in the least painful way. One of the reasons why so many British childcare experts insist that children under three are incapable of making friendships, and disturbed by leaving their mothers, is probably because they are looking at kids who are rarely separated and likely to be left in unfamiliar circumstances with unfamiliar people. Professor Barbara Tizard, Director of the Thomas Coram Unit at the Institute of Education, has this to say about irregular arrangements for under-threes:

'The need to maintain constancy amongst the children in a group has received little attention. . . . The research suggests that simply bringing unfamiliar children together is of very limited benefit to them. For this reason "Drop In Centres", or mother and toddler clubs where the child population is constantly changing, have relatively little to offer children.'

Of course these clubs can have enormous value for parents or child carers bringing up children in very isolated and cramped conditions, as they provide more space and different experiences for young children to investigate and companionship for adults. However they do not, as Tizard points out, provide an isolated child with friends unless deliberate attempts are made to encourage relationships on a regular basis.

If you arrange swops, or want to leave your child to play with a friend occasionally, it helps to visit with her the first time. Don't wait for an emergency when you are forced to drop her off and then escape as fast as possible. If we want our children to regard visits to friends as treats rather than traumas they need to experience them that way.

IF YOUR CHILD IS UNHAPPY

If your child is very distressed about being left, and does not start to settle, try to work out why *before* you make any decision about changing the situation. It may be that the care you have chosen is unsatisfactory but, if there is some other reason, you will do more harm than good by moving him so that he has to go through the difficulty of adjusting all over again in a new situation.

SHARING FEEDING

Being able to share feeding with another person is vital if you are to share care for more than very short periods. This is no problem for bottle-feeding parents:

'Being so tied to the first two I found the bottle very liberating. Once I had got over the trauma it was wonderful. I could go out and know that the child wasn't hungry if I got stuck in a traffic jam.'

Many mothers going back to work find that it is very hard indeed to wean their babies off the breast and on to a bottle during the day. In most cases, left with another person, babies will eventually take to bottle feeds but Geraldine found that, at four months:

'She refuses to take any liquid during the day and wakes up every four hours at night instead. I am not worrying about it because she is taking solid food and throughout the day she gets enough of everything, but I am getting very tired.'

If you intend to leave your baby with anyone else during the first months it helps to introduce a bottle early even if you only use it for water or very dilute fruit juice. This way your baby will get used to the idea of a bottle at a time when its use is not also associated with the stress of losing you.

You can also express your own milk using a breast pump (available in chemists) and then either leave it in the fridge or freeze it for use by babysitters or your partner. However you do have to take the same hygiene precautions as any other bottle feeder (see Chapter 8). I know of some women who have shared feeding with partners throughout the early months this way. Vincent remembers:

'I wanted to have her on my own for a night. She was about six weeks the first time. I had a bottle of expressed milk and she hated bottles, but she woke and had it that night and then I had nothing to give her in the morning. The bottle became a big thing. Once it took 1½ hours to give her a feed. It was a hassle but it was worth it in the end.'

However we don't all find expressing that easy:

'I felt like a cow. Sitting at the kitchen table with a pump on my breast. It was uncomfortable, laborious and it would take about half an hour to squeeze out an ounce. With my second child I didn't even try. I just decided that, for four months, I would keep her

with me. It meant I couldn't go to the cinema but it seemed a pretty small price to pay.'

Doubling up with other lactating mothers provides not only company and support but also a back-up food supply. For occasional babysitting such an arrangement can be a real boon although, as one mother said:

'There was something rather strange about it at first. It took me back to the feeling I had with a new boyfriend when I was very young.'

Midwives Janet and Jane lived together so they were able to feed each other's babies and provide each other with child care to fit in with their shifts:

'I fed Nell at least once a day for about five days out of seven. I always had masses of milk and was never engorged until I tried to wean my own child. They were both quite clear who their own mothers were. I suppose confusion could arise if they had absolutely equal handling as well as inter-changeable breastfeeding but it wasn't like that.'

Sharing on this intimate level provides the children with an enormous amount of security but it is pretty tiring for the mothers involved:

'If you were not working you were coping with two children. There never seemed to be any break.'

Some women returning to work in the first six months continue to express milk at work, refrigerate it, and then leave it for the baby's feeds the next day. This is certainly a feasible option for anyone who has a copious milk supply and is particularly concerned about introducing other kinds of milk in the early months (see Chapter 5). However, it is not necessary to keep on expressing by day simply in order to keep up your milk supply for evening feeds. Your body will very quickly adjust to producing the amount of milk your baby is actually taking. At this stage you can introduce formula milk or rely on solid food and very dilute fruit juice to provide calories and liquid, and then make sure the baby gets plenty of milk from you in the evening. In fact you will do more to maintain your milk supply by using your lunch break to relax and feed yourself than by spending it frantically trying to squeeze out a few ounces of milk while sitting perched on a toilet in a cold loo!

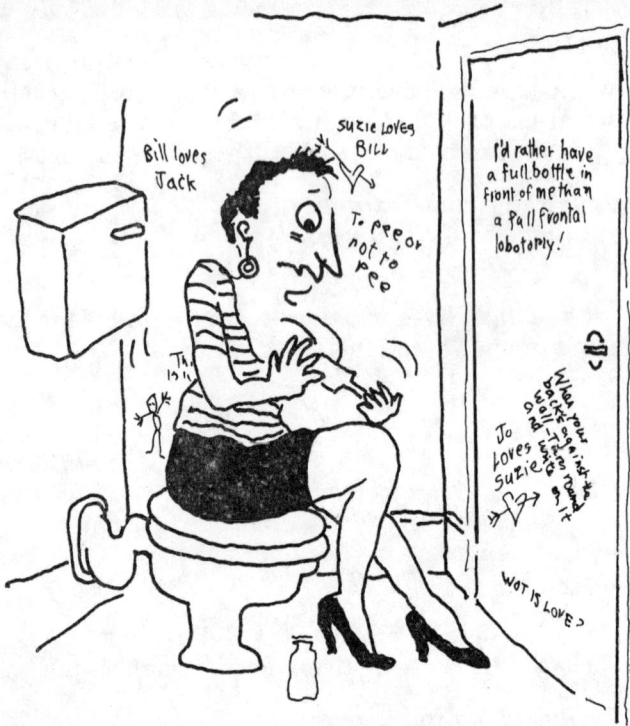

It might help to consider your own feelings first. Children do react differently to being left but so do their mothers. This quote from a nursery teacher, passed on by Bettleheim in his book *The Good Enough Parent*, may help to put it in perspective:

'In this teacher's experience, only those children whose mothers have a difficult time separating from them have a difficult time themselves separating from their mothers. A mother who truly feels that nursery school will be good for her child conveys this message through her behaviour. She leaves the child on the first day at school without much hesitation, and he is soon happily engaged in activity. The story is quite the opposite if a parent has inner doubts about leaving a child; she conveys this by lingering on, making a move to leave only to return immediately at the first sign of uneasiness on the part of the child. Soon the child senses that his mother thinks that leaving him is not a good thing so he begins to cry and hang on to her.'

If your feelings about leaving your child are ambivalent you would not be the first! Try to consider honestly (maybe a friend could help) whether you are really confident about where, and with whom you are leaving your child.

If you are not confident in your carer you cannot make your child feel confident. If you feel that the place and people are not the problem then you need to work on your own feelings.

Don't expect miracles. Some children may be very unsettled for the first week or two. If you are still concerned, talk to your carer. Does your child settle quickly (within ten minutes) when you leave? Is he happy during the day? Is he getting a sleep when he needs it? Does he have the things he needs to feel secure (his special blanket, bottle or dummy)? It is not a good idea to try and break a child of a comfort habit when he is just starting in a new place unless he has decided to make the break himself.

Perhaps his other parent or a close friend could take him in for a few days. If the misery is about leaving you rather than going to the new person, it won't be hard to find out. He will still cry on leaving you but may be very happy to see his day carer. If you are still uncertain about the care situation, try making a few spot checks during the day to see if he is happy and well cared for. If your child is old enough to talk about it, encourage him to do so, but don't interrogate him – you may be transmitting your own anxiety. Watch out also for other signs of distress such as bedwetting or nightmares. They don't necessarily mean any more than that your child is reacting to a change of circumstances, but some extra reassurance from you won't go amiss.

If you are convinced that the situation itself is upsetting him, start looking for something else but move cautiously. If you rush you may end up with something worse and then have to disrupt him again. Read the next section on making choices. Remember that it is you who must feel happy about child care if your child is to feel happy too. Don't leave him with people you do not trust. When you do find a carer that you trust, give them a chance to form a relationship before you make judgements.

If you suspect that your child is being abused or mistreated you cannot just wait and see – you will have to remove him at once and make other arrangements. Always notify the Social Services department of your suspicions. They register child carers and should investigate any such complaints in order to protect others.

FINDING CHILDCARE

Few of us have the money to be able to make real decisions about child care. On the whole we have to take the best of what is available within our price range. However it is worth thinking through the various options so that we can work out our priorities, even if we fail to fulfil them.

Whatever child care we choose it is important that it provides all the things that children need: secure attachments to responsive carers, opportunities to get to know other children; a safe and healthy environment; good food; stimulating play at a level they are ready for; the opportunity to sleep when they need to. Once these needs are satisfied our decisions depend very much on our own gut feelings, our own experience, and our own preferences. If we do not satisfy *ourselves* about child care we will never be able to leave our children without worrying about them.

Individual or group care?

This is the first decision. Research in Scandinavia and in Belgium has compared different kinds of care and come to the conclusion that, as long as the children's basic needs are provided for, there is no difference in outcome whether they are in group or individual care. So try to think about what you want and what is available.

Are you looking for a replacement mother or someone/some people to supplement your own mothering? Or a combination of the two? Much depends on whether this will be fulltime care for nine or ten hours a day for a baby or a few hours every morning for a two-year-old. Susha needed fulltime care for two children both under three:

> 'The ideal for me would be to have them in a small group when they are not with me so that I can feel they are really getting something different.'

Since her working hours are erratic and often long, she compromised with a nanny to provide basic care and a small group once a week (at eighteen months), playgroup in the mornings (at two years) and finally day nursery for the older child at nearly three.

Babies
In the first year of life many parents opt for care with a childminder or nanny to ensure that the baby will get plenty of individual attention and handling, as well as being able to sleep when necessary. If you are sharing a nanny make sure she can confidently handle more than one baby. Otherwise it may be easier to share with an older child. This mother opted for a nursery because she felt hopeless about judging the abilities of an individual carer. Nevertheless, in retrospect she says:

> 'I do still have doubts about group care for under two's. She found the noise level difficult and was excessively shy for a while. She went through a very bad patch of howling all day when she had apparently been settled.'

Susan was absolutely clear about wanting a nursery rather than individual care:

'I would be concerned about leaving my baby with someone unsupervised who I didn't know well. Having him in a workplace nursery means that I can visit him at lunch time and I know exactly what is happening, where he is going, and what he is eating. There is a clear policy.'

Toddlers and pre-school children

After the first year there is plenty of evidence that children thrive on the regular company of others. They may not be immediately ready to play together at this age but they are ready to start making relationships and, if they see the same children regularly, those children become part of their lives. They provide each other with security in much the same way as with another familiar adult.

'Our children love one another. Not like brothers and sisters – they rarely fight. There is an equality about it, and a contentment with each other's company, as well as a real concern and affection which is wonderful to witness.'

If, for example, you opt for a nanny to look after your child alone, when that nanny leaves your child will have to start all over again with someone new. If your child is being cared for with another child their friendship will be some protection against the loss. Sharing a nanny is not just a way of sharing costs – it benefits the children.

Similarly, in a nursery, provided that children are cared for in stable groups where they can build up close relationships with other children, there will be a measure of protection when the carer changes. With a childminder you will not get that protection. Professor Barbara Tizard comments:

'Unstable childminding is notoriously disturbing to children; at each change the child must adjust not only to a new childminder but also to a new house, and new child companions.'

This does not mean that childminders cannot provide good care but it is wise to try and get some idea of how long your minder intends to stay with the job, and to find someone who can accommodate your needs easily. If you have to persuade your carer, for example, to keep the child an hour later than she really wants you may be building in a problem for the future.

What to look for

Caring carers

You may know nothing about child care or what to expect from a carer but you have not completely lost your sense of judgement about other people

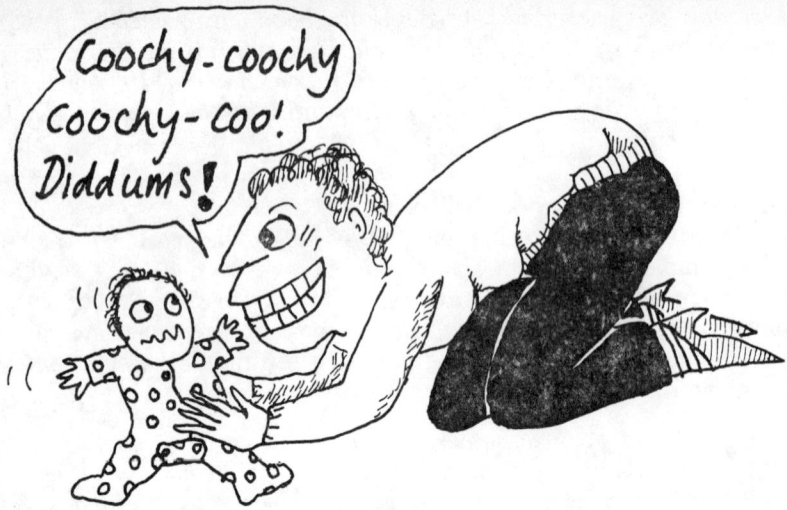

simply as people. In the end, it will be the quality of that person's ability to care which will really count.

'I nearly left John with some pretty hopeless people. Then I found
Susan through an ad in the local paper. As we talked, she had her
own baby on her knee. She continually caressed her, talked lovingly to
her and never stopped being "with" her baby, in order to talk to me.
I just knew that this was a person with a big enough capacity to love.
She would love my kid too even if he was unbearable at times.'

Probably the best way to judge a good childminder is to see her with her own children. If the children are older, try to visit after school. Don't be put off if they seem enormous and noisy compared to your child. You want to see if they are happy and whether they are allowed to feel free in their own home. If they show a friendly interest in your child that is an added bonus.

If you are interviewing a nanny try to give her (or him) some time with your child. You can move aside to make tea or invent an urgent phonecall (you don't have to leave the room). Does she immediately go to the child's level, engage directly, talk (even to a small baby)? Someone who really understands about small children will be careful not to move in too close, too fast, and alarm them, but will not ignore them either.

If you are visiting a nursery you need to know how many children are being cared for and how many adults are directly involved in their care. Local authorities usually demand one adult to every two or three babies (under twos) and one adult to every four or five over that age. Find out how babies are cared for (if this is relevant). Is there a special room or do they have a 'key worker' scheme with one or two workers specially responsible for each baby but working also with older children? Are the children looked after in small groups with one person in charge, or allowed to move freely around the place between different activities? Is there a conscious effort to allow children to become attached to one or two workers and to other children? Is there a high staff turnover? Above all, are the children happy? If you think they are unhappy, don't send your child there.

In all cases get references or try to find out what other parents think of your potential carer. Talk to health visitors and council Under Fives workers too.

Shared values

This will help to provide a harmonious arrangement. Black parents will want to be particularly careful about their choice of carer. A carer may be just as loving to the black children in her care as she is to the white children. Nevertheless she may be expecting her charges to conform entirely to her own value system. She may automatically speak of white as good (the white fairy) and black as bad (the black witch). A child's confidence is rooted on feeling good about herself, her family and her culture. Her carers should reflect her own background and its values back to her in a way which will allow her to feel positive about them. Simply having other black adults and children around will help.

'We started off with four white children and one black in our group. Then a second black child joined. These two children did not make a stronger relationship with each other but Josephine would always ask for Adil if he was late in the morning. She just liked to know he was there.'

All children start off with a positive attitude to themselves and to others. A white child is curious about black skin but sees it only as another variation. It is we adults who inject values in the way we talk about other people. In these early years our children are starting to form their view of the world. It is up to the adults in their lives to ensure that they learn to value each other's cultures and to learn about each other's lives.

If a black child is to grow up proud and strong she must grow up with a positive reflection of her blackness. If a white child is to grow up rejecting the racism which is so deeply embedded in white society she too needs to grow up with a positive reflection of blackness. Anti-racist child care is for all our children.

Some councils provide equal opportunities training for all under-fives workers in the borough. Contact your local Social Services department to find out if they have taken up this issue and can refer you to child carers with equal opportunity training. Failing that, you could start by asking your carer if you can provide some books and puzzles with pictures of black children, and explain why it is important to you.

Similarly, make sure you and your carer agree about things like discipline. If you never smack your child and don't want anyone else to, say so. Don't assume anything.

A safe and healthy environment

This is obviously something you will be concerned about. For many children, the hours in day care are longer than the waking hours at home. You should insist on a high standard. If you live in cramped conditions with no outside space your child should be given the advantage of a better place to spend the day. If you live in a large house with a garden, do you want your child to be spending most of her time in conditions worse than she would have at home?

You also have a right to insist that your child gets regular fresh air and exercise. If your potential carer lives in a flat without a garden she may still be a wonderful minder, but you should ensure that she is prepared to take your child to the park and on visits to One O'Clock Clubs or toddler groups where there is more space.

Are there opportunities for your child to sleep when she needs to? An energetic carer who is out and about all day may seem wonderful but a two-year-old may prefer the peace of spending a good portion of every day in a familiar and restful place. Nurseries, minders or nannies all need to be prepared to take a child's individual need for sleep into consideration. If they don't you will wind up with a tired, miserable child to come home to. A child can usually adapt quite quickly to sleeping at a convenient time but will get very ratty if the amount of sleep she needs is restricted.

Check the noise level. Some nurseries are very noisy and that can be hard, specially for a small child. Find out if there is a 'quiet room' or periods of the day when quiet activities are imposed so that all the children get some rest.

Is there a healthy diet? If your child goes to a nursery check in advance what kind of food policy they have. Good food policies are much more common than they were. If your nursery doesn't have one, get together with other parents and see if you can draw one up. If you have a nanny you will be providing the food but you won't be there to see how it's prepared. Be clear about what you want your child to eat but keep it simple. It is hard work preparing food while you are looking after small children and you are not paying her to be a cook.

Suitable stimulation

We don't all expect our children to be Einstein's but most of us want them to fulfil their own potential. Probably the most important thing your child needs is someone around who will talk to her rather than shoving her in front of the TV. Try to get an opportunity to observe your carer with children. Does she communicate directly with the child or only with you? Are there toys around? Will your child be able to make a mess? If your carer's house is very tidy ask where, and when, your child would be able to handle messy things like paint, water or play dough. Will your child be taken out to suitable places such as One O' Clock Clubs, toy libraries or toddler groups? Will she ensure that your child has regular contact with other children and is able to build up friendships? You may want to combine an individual carer with a playgroup or school nursery, in which case make sure your name is on all relevant waiting lists.

Establishing a contract

Mothers often express concern about dealing, as an employer, with an individual. Shusha said:

> 'It's pretty awkward having a "servant". It doesn't make it easy to discuss things, it's so personal. In my own home I want to control everything and yet I don't want to be oppressive of the other woman. So I don't know what to say.'

Other people prefer nannies just because they feel they *can* have total control. Of course this is a myth. If you are not there you cannot control your nanny's behaviour. Indeed, it is only by fostering a really trusting relationship and encouraging your nanny to share in decision-making about child care that you are likely to get her to tell you what is really going on. If your child is screaming for two hours every morning when you leave, or beating up the other children at the drop-in centre, it takes a fairly confident nanny to discuss it with you, in case you blame her.

The same problems can occur with a childminder except that in her own home and (usually) with some experience of parenting she doesn't feel at such a disadvantage – she is offering a service and she is definitely not your servant. Many parents are glad of another, more experienced, person to seek advice from. In an ideal situation parents and minder feel that they are partners looking after children they all care about. In this atmosphere of personal trust it should be easy to discuss problems.

Whoever is caring for your child, you need to make sure that you are both clear about what is expected – on both sides. If your child is going to a nursery ask about the nursery policy on issues that concern you. Are parents involved in the management of the nursery (if not, why not)? Is there an anti-racist policy? Is the nursery consciously non-sexist in its treatment of girls and boys? Are there regular open evenings so that you can discuss your child's progress? What kinds of records are kept? If you have an individual carer make sure they understand exactly what you want (and don't want). In all cases write down anything which is particularly important: diet; sleep;

care of such things as skin conditions or asthma. Rules may seem fierce but can make things much clearer for someone working in your home.

Make sure that your movements are clear and that everyone knows when you will drop the child off and pick her up. It is irritating to wait for a child who comes late and it can disrupt the day for any other children involved. If there are occasions when you are likely to be late collecting say so in advance. Your carer has a right to her own life whether in your home or her own.

Check on holiday arrangements in advance. Nurseries may have a closed period in the summer. Your nanny or minder will want to make her own arrangements too.

Make sure you understand how much money you are expected to pay, your obligations regarding National Insurance and Tax, and what arrangements will be made during holidays and periods of sickness.

If you are employing a nanny keep in mind the fact that looking after small children is extremely demanding and often very isolated work. Make sure your nanny is certain she wants this sort of life. Try to help her to meet other nannies in the area or to attend a nanny group. (If there aren't any perhaps you could start one.) If you want her to care happily for your children you must care well enough for her to ensure that she is happy too.

It is worth getting information from the National Childminding Association about a contract with your minder. The Working Mothers Association has a 'nanny pack' for the employers of nannies (see p. 211).

WHERE TO FIND CARE

Start well in advance of returning to work. Go first to your local council, who should have a list of all registered childminders and nurseries.

Nurseries

There is a shortage of reasonably priced, good quality care of any kind, but a chronic shortage of nurseries. What there is is divided between council nurseries (nearly always reserved only for children at risk but occasionally also for single parents), voluntary (or community) nurseries which may be subsidised by the council but will have massive waiting lists, and private nurseries which rarely take children under two years old and charge very high rates if they do.

There are also a few workplace nurseries, and it seems likely that these facilities will increase over the next few years. Unfortunately, at the time of writing, the government has refused to waive the tax on any childcare subsidy paid by employers. The cost of tax, on top of nursery fees, means that even subsidised workplace provision is not cheap enough for many people on average incomes.

All nurseries must be registered and should, therefore, be on the council list. Nurseries rarely have immediate vacancies but most will have waiting lists and you should get your name down as early as possible if you are interested in nursery care.

Playgroups and nursery classes

These usually only run for 2½ hours a day. If you are at home, or have a childminder or nanny, you will want to get on these lists too. Contact your local Preschool Playgroups Association (look in the phone book), visit schools in your area to look at their nurseries and talk to other parents for recommendations. Put your name on lists as soon as possible.

Childminders

Some councils will give you a list and expect you to get on and contact everyone on it. Others will give you names of minders with vacancies. At the time of writing there was a shortage of minders and some councils had simply stopped referring parents who were not in pretty desperate circumstances. Ask about your council's service. Do they regularly visit childminders and supply support in the form of minders' groups, training or a toy library? Many councils do nothing more than inspect for safety problems and drop in once every couple of years to see if the minder wants to keep her name on a list. Registration does *not* imply a recommendation. The best childminders may circulate by word of mouth. Tell everyone you can think of that you will be needing care well in advance and advertise locally.

Nannies

Nannies are unregistered, unregulated and responsible only to you. You can employ someone who doesn't know one end of a baby from the other – it's up to you. You may want to go through a nanny agency (though this will almost certainly cost a lot more), or through advertising in *The Lady* or *Nursery World*. You could also try advertising locally in shop windows, your local paper, etc. If you want to share a nanny with another family contact a nanny share register (your local National Childbirth Trust or Working Mothers Association groups will know if there is one locally), or advertise in shop windows, on health centre notice boards, etc. Once you find a compatible family you can look for a nanny together.

If you work full time look for someone who is either qualified or very experienced. The nursery nurse qualification (for 0–5s) is an NNEB, and the Preschool Playgroups Association does PPA training for people working with toddlers and pre-schoolers. A nursing training is also relevant, at least for babies. If you are considering an untrained nanny, an experienced child-minder or a woman who has brought up her own family will at least know exactly what she is letting herself in for and should be able to cope with tantrums, tears and the difficult moments when a young, inexperienced girl may feel inclined to lash out or walk out. If you only want care for a few hours a week a less experienced person can probably cope.

Doing it yourself

Swopping
If you work part time or job share you may want to consider doubling up with another mother and sharing child care between you. This can work pretty well if you like looking after children, but as a form of regular care it is extremely tiring and isolating and leaves you with no time to spend alone with your child. You may also have to cope with your own child's jealousy at having your time and attention diverted. This can result in some displays of extremely demanding behaviour.

'Sharing child care with a good friend was one of the worst things I remember about early parenthood. It had sounded easy – and of course very cheap but I had little experience of caring for children other than my own and was shocked to discover how hard, unrewarding and plain boring it was. Our children were just over a year old. Her child was very unsettled and cried a lot. After a while, mine became angry and jealous because of the attention she was getting. He took it out on her rather than me and she started crying whenever she saw him. I might have coped if I hadn't had the additional pressure of my own work to deal with. I was either coping with two fractious kids or frantically trying to earn a living – there was no respite.'

By the time your child is nursery age, short, regular swops can work well because the children will be relating mainly to each other rather than competing for you. It also helps children to build close friendships which can be a great help when starting school.

Parent coops
These may be a positive solution or just a stop-gap response to the child care shortage. They can be organised in a number of ways.

A group of, say, six parents can get together and devise a rota so that, in pairs, they look after all the children together. Parents provide each other with company and support for the day on and get a couple of free days knowing that their children are being equally well cared for by other parents. These groups are better kept small because it is hard for children to get used to more than six constantly changing caretakers.

Another model involves a group of at least five parents employing a worker between them and then spending a day each a week working along-side her with the children. This model allows parents four free days and ensures that the worker can be paid at a reasonable hourly rate because her wages are shared.

Fulltime working parents can easily set up a group of this kind by employing two workers between, for example, five families. This ensures that the workers are not isolated and the children have regular companions whom they can get to know well. The five sets of parents can then provide back-up in case of staff illness.

Most of these groups are run in private homes, but a few have managed to find accommodation in public buildings: schools, libraries, etc. It is worth approaching your local council, education authority and individual schools, to ask if there is any available and suitable space. If you use public property you should be registered by the council.

All these solutions require a high level of organisation and communi-cation between parents and workers. Regular meetings are essential. If the groups are run on public property they should be accountable to the com-munity. That means allowing access to parents who are not part of your immediate circle. If you have big enough homes to run a group in you will probably avoid the legal need to be registered but you will have to cope with a high level of mess and disruption. If you move the crêche around to different houses your children will have to get used to a constantly changing environment as well as a variety of carers, which can be hard on them. In spite of the difficulties involved in managing a parent-run crêche, the advantages are enormous. You have the opportunity of actually participating in your childs' day care and getting to know a number of other children very well.

CHANGING WORK

Women in the UK, more than most other countries, tend to leave their jobs when the first baby arrives and then go back to another job at a lower level of pay and skill. The major reason for this drop in status is not our lack of interest in the world of work but the inability of that male-dominated world to take into consideration our needs and the needs of our children.

Sadly, most male parents collude in this child-blindness. They go along with the rules, often work long hours, and make it impossible not only for them to form meaningful relationships with their own children, or help out at home, but also for their partners to take on a more responsible job. When it comes to the crunch someone has to stay at home when Johnny has measles, be there to read bedtime stories, or hear about the first day at nursery. That someone is nearly always Mum, so it is Mum who is forced to drop out and go part-time.

This does not need to be so. Even in the most high-powered jobs there is room for some adjustment. Perhaps a News Editor cannot work a six-hour day in order to be home to put the kids to bed, but there is no God-given reason why he and his partner cannot each work a four-day week. This work pattern would allow each partner to work impossible shifts – if there is a crying need for it – and at the same time ensure that the children only have to be cared for by another person for three days in a week. Most kids could cope with someone else tucking them into bed two or three nights a week if Mum or Dad are around to care for them the other four. Vince changed his work time to share the care of his daughter.

'I took a day off every week for two years. We doubled up with another family and three of us looked after two babies for a day a week. It was very hard work but I did it because I wanted to and because I had a job which allowed me to.'

Some partners working in similar jobs have been able to job-share in order to ensure that both of them keep a toe in the labour market and on the career ladder for the first few years. That way the children get plenty of parent care and neither parent is disadvantaged in the job market. These models have not changed the face of work as we know it, but they do indicate ways for the future. For the present many of us are lumbered with trying to decide what compromises we can afford to make.

Susha has a demanding, high-paying job in television, and a partner with an equally demanding job who is not inclined to share the care of two small children. She says:

'I do think full-time high pressure work and small children don't mix. I could also say that I've been lucky. I have a flexible job. I've kept my feet under the desk and I get variety, prestige and money.'

Her 'luck' was to have an employer who recognised her dilemma and proposed a short-term solution. She was asked if she would like to return to work to what was essentially a desk job for six months. That would give the children time to get used to their new carer and give her time to work out what she could manage. Now, with one three-year-old child and another of eighteen months, she is back on the production side:

'They are flourishing. I don't feel guilty but I do regret not seeing even more of them than I do.'

She still manages to see as much of them as her schedule allows and is very strict about taking time off in lieu that is due to her when she has been working away, but she rarely feels able to so 'officially'. Indeed, she refers to it as 'skiving'. She will probably continue to slip off early without drawing attention to herself because it is very hard for a mother in our society to stand up and say: 'I am leaving early because I have finished my work and I want to see my children.' Leaving early (or even promptly) is seen as evidence of a shaky commitment to work. As Sandra, a trade union officer, says:

> 'If men say they are not available at a certain time it's OK. If a mother says it she's incompetent. It is very important that working fathers take on the arguments and don't leave women to fight alone.'

Changing working schedules is hard if you are on your own. It's a great deal easier if people higher up the department take on some of the battles for you. Jess, a single parent, is an assistant department director for a Labour Local Authority.

> 'When I took the job I said that I couldn't start until 9.30 in the morning. I was determined to be able to take my child to school in the morning myself. It was particularly important because I often have to work late in the afternoon. For the first few weeks they went on organising departmental meetings at 8.30. I just didn't attend and in the end they got the message that I meant what I said.'

When Josie landed a new job she insisted on taking an afternoon off a week in order to be with her children.

> 'In my previous job I had bargained for a few hours off on Thursday afternoon in return for working late another day. This time, going for a new job, I had the confidence just to ask for the time off without making compromises. They wanted me so they agreed.'

For parents with less power there is very little flexibility. Lynette wanted to join a parent-run crêche, spending one day a week with the children, and working a six-hour day, four days a week. There was plenty of part-time work available but nothing fitting that shift pattern and no one ready to make any compromises.

We are a very long way away from the Swedish solution to the conflicts between work and child care. In Sweden parents have a statutory right to work a six-hour day until their children start school, at seven years old. It is a solution which allows both parents to stay on a career path while at the same time taking joint responsibility for providing that 'quality time'. In Scandinavia fathers are also positively encouraged to take paternity leave. It is generally assumed that both men and women will work and it is the responsibility of the government and employers to ease working schedules so that children will not lose out. A long way to go maybe – but worth fighting for.

Chapter 8

HEALTH AND SAFETY

Christopher Robin
Got up in the morning
The sneezles had vanished away
And the look in his eye
Seemed to say to the sky
'Now, how to amuse them to-day?'
(A. A. Milne, *Now We Are Six*)

During pregnancy your baby has been kept at exactly the right temperature, fed automatically, cushioned and rocked in a soft and sterile environment. Short of keeping well yourself you have not had to do anything to help this process. Once the baby is outside all these automatic processes suddenly become responsibilities.

'She seemed so small it was impossible to imagine that she could survive. When she slept her breathing was so light that sometimes I would prod her a little to make her stir – just to reassure myself that she was actually breathing.'

A basic understanding of health care for babies and young children covers four areas: 1) how to build up their own resistance to disease; 2) how to protect them from organisms which may make them ill and accidents which can hurt them; 3) how to deal with minor health problems; 4) how to decide where our own experience ends and when we need professional help.

Your child's best protection against disease is her own body, which is equipped with a far more sophisticated defence and attack system than any doctor can provide. As parents we can help our children build up their natural resistance by feeding them well (see Chapter 5) and making sure they have as much opportunity as they need for exercise and sleep, stimulation and peace.

General good health will help your child fight diseases but it won't stop him from getting them. Each time your child gets ill, he is building up his immune system which in turn provides protection against disease the next time it strikes. This protection is so good that, in the case of some of the

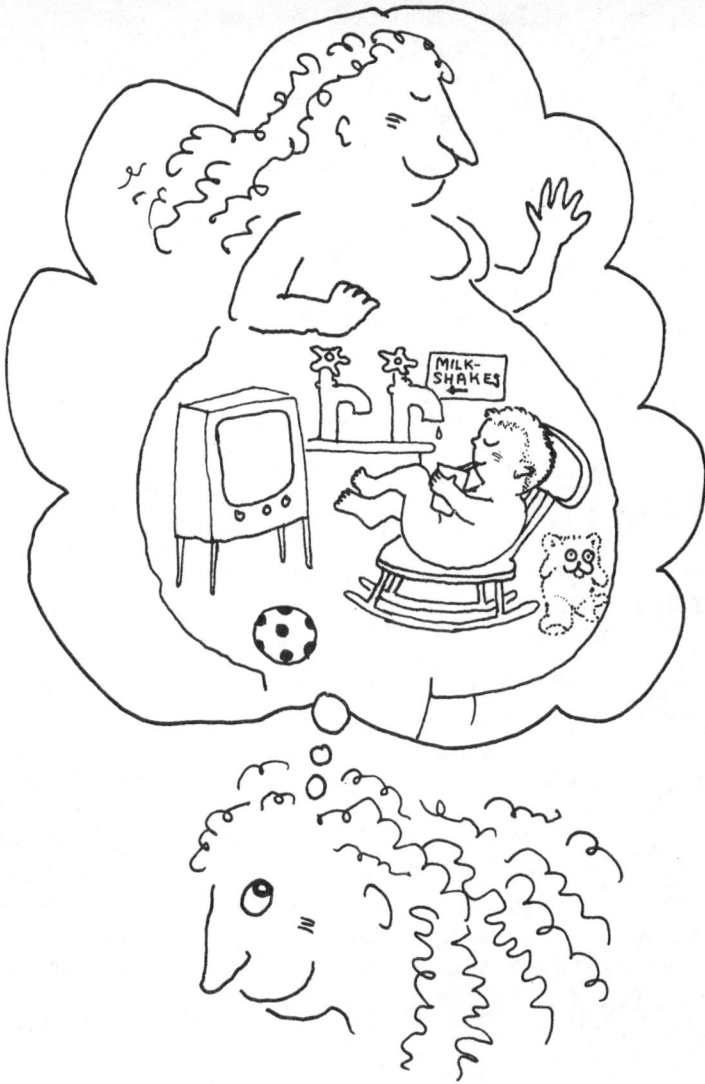

most serious infectious diseases, the first attack provides total immunity. The child will never get that disease again.

Immunisation is a way of stimulating your childs defences against these diseases *before* they strike. Most parents choose to take advantage of innoculation against the major infectious diseases of childhood: Diptheria, Tetanus, Polio and Whooping Cough (a series of three innoculations in the first year), and Measles, Rubella and Mumps (in the second year). In some areas

Tuberculosis protection will be offered too. Booster immunization is offered just before the child starts school.

If your child is being cared for with other children, most carers will insist on immunisation to keep down the level of infection. If you are looking after your child at home, you may prefer to let him go through the disease himself. However, if you do, you must take responsibility for the possibility that your child could infect another child, who may not be as healthy as yours and could get very ill indeed. Although immunisation is an individual decision, lack of immunisation does not have an individual effect. Only by mass immunisation have we managed to virtually erradicate killer diseases like polio and diptheria. If large numbers of parents had decided to opt out of these programmes our children would be at much higher risk today.

A mild fever and some grouchiness is a pretty common side effect some time within the twenty-four hours following the jab. If your baby has a history of convulsions, or reacts severely to the first shot, it may be better to avoid the whooping cough element of the triple vaccine as there is a small risk of a serious reaction.

A GUIDE TO GOOD HEALTH

Hot or cold

Babies find it difficult to regulate their own temperature. They can very easily become overheated or chilled if we do not take care to keep them at a reasonable temperature. Aim to keep room temperatures at about 65°F (18°C) night and day. Be just as careful to avoid *overheating*. If your baby is getting sweaty at night he may be overwrapped, which can force his temperature up to dangerous levels. Keep night clothing light (a single stretch suit will do). In the first three months it is best to provide warmth through layers of cellular blankets. This way air can still circulate around the baby's body. While sleeping your baby does not need to be any warmer than you are in bed. When out of the cot it may help to think in terms of one layer more than you are wearing to make up for the fact that the baby is not moving much.

Once your child is moving around easily keeping the temperature right is no longer such a problem. Crawling babies and toddlers create their own heat. At night your major problem may be to keep the child covered at all. This is not likely to be a threat to health (they wake up when they get cold) – however, it might be a threat to your sleep! A very wriggly older baby or child may sleep better in a zip-up warm sleep suit. Do not put more than a vest on underneath it or you may again be trapping far too much heat against the skin.

Out of doors, children who run about seem to cope with getting thoroughly chilled without any ill effect. The problem is often to persuade them to keep enough clothing on for our peace of mind. If they are moving freely they are almost certainly keeping themselves warm. They need more care in the sun. Babies should never be left in direct sunshine and older children are better off playing in light shade on a sunny day with short bursts of sun. On a beach, it is wise to encourage children to wear their hats, and to limit exposure until they have started to get used to the sun. White children should always have a high protection factor sunscreen for exposed skin. Make sure your children have plenty to drink.

If your child starts to feel sick or complains of a headache, get him out of the sun, give him a cool drink, and gently cool him down. Heat stroke can be dangerous. If the child's temperature starts to shoot up alarmingly in spite of attempts to cool her down, contact your doctor straight away, or take the child to a hospital.

Clean dirt and dirty dirt

Our grandmothers (or great grandmothers) knew a great deal about hygiene. They knew that if you didn't keep things clean or eat food fresh then people would get ill and, without the help of antibiotics, these illnesses could be very serious indeed, particularly for young children. We have stopped paying much attention to hygiene because we live in a world in which we assume that it is taken care of by modern conveniences such as built-in kitchens, bottles of liquids for killing germs, and food which comes clean and packaged out of one refrigerator into another. Nevertheless, in order to protect babies and small children, we do need to take extra precautions. That doesn't mean becoming a fanatical house-cleaner. It means knowing the difference between clean dirt and dirty dirt.

Splashes of paint, the general stains of life and living are not a health hazard. You do not need to wash the floor frantically and clean the skirting boards when your child learns to crawl. A two-year-old who has paint stains all over her hands, mud under her finger nails, and sand in her hair has clearly been having a good time exploring her environment. Auntie might object to what she looks like but this kind of dirt is not a health hazard.

Dirty dirt is the kind that breeds bacteria, and bacteria can cause infection if they get into a cut or are swallowed. We all have our own built-in protection against infection. That resistance is built up by gradual exposure to small amounts of bacteria. A newborn baby will get ill if only a small amount of harmful bacteria gets into his system. A toddler has already built up enough resistance to deal with many of the dubious things she is likely to find and put in her mouth. The best way to protect her from harm is to ensure that harmful bacteria are kept to a minimum so that she can never take in enough to overwhelm her defences.

Bacteria live all over and inside any organic matter (anything animal or vegetable, alive or dead). Some are extremely harmful, others do little damage in small quantities and some are positively useful. The important thing is to prevent the bad ones from multiplying and keep the good ones in useful balance. In a healthy, living organism, good bacteria live in balance with bad bacteria and keep them from multiplying out of proportion. If the bad ones overgrow and crowd out the good ones you will get ill.

Bacteria grow and thrive on dead matter, particularly if it is left in warm, wet places. They do not like very cold or very hot temperatures. Food that is left around, dirty nappies, open bottles of milk all provide breeding points for harmful bacteria. Bottles, teats and feeder beaker tops provide lots of crevices where bits of food can collect.

Clean cups, plates, spoons, clothes and other baby equipment do not provide a happy breeding ground. It is perfectly safe to give medicine to a baby off a clean, dry spoon which has been sitting in a drawer, but less safe to give it off a newly washed spoon which is then wiped with a damp drying-up cloth. The damp cloth can harbour bacteria – the dry spoon won't. Similarly if a plastic toy falls on a recently washed kitchen floor it can be given back. There has been no opportunity for bacteria to be picked up. If it falls on the street (or in the toilet) it should be well washed first.

Keeping it clean

Waste products

These should be kept well away from your baby and from uneaten food. Your baby's own waste products can be a source of infection if they are not dealt with properly. Pee, when it comes out, is usually sterile. If there is a puddle on the floor, just mop it up. However, wet nappies which are not washed or disposed of immediately can provide a breeding ground for bacteria from elsewhere.

Soiled nappies are already full of bacteria which will multiply fast. It is best to flush the solid stuff down the toilet (if necessary by tearing off the top layer of a disposable nappy). Then put all nappies into a covered bin until you can dispose of them or sterilise them.

Dirty nappies should be kept well away from food and you should always wash your hands thoroughly after nappy changing. A speck of baby shit under a fingernail can be very easily transferred to food being prepared. If you are caring for more than one child these things are even more important as gastro-enteritis (diarrhoea and vomiting) can be passed from one child to another.

Toilets should be kept shit free and toilet brushes should be rinsed well as you flush, and then kept well away from small children. Surfaces which are used for eating or preparing food need to be washed down regularly. You don't need to use chemicals. Just make sure blobs of butter or gravy do not set up germ factories.

Food waste should not be left where a young child may be able to help herself and cat litter trays should be regularly changed and cleaned, kept out of eating areas, and away from small children.

Breasts and bodies

These present no threat to your baby. Babies build resistance not only by drinking their mother's milk but also by gradually getting used to the small amounts of bacteria that live on clean skin. That said, anyone handling a baby should take care to wash their own hands after going to the toilet, or after handling raw meat.

Small children have their hands in their mouths much of the time so it is very hard to stop them swallowing, for example, lead-filled dirt from an urban park. Hand-washing will keep the dirt level down but not completely out. Do be very careful to wash hands as fast as possible if a child inadvertently picks up dog shit. It is teeming with bacteria and should not be allowed in the mouth, eyes (or children's areas or parks) at all.

Daily bathing is a good idea for children who are out of nappies but not yet very good at wiping themselves. Urine and shit which is not properly cleaned off can cause irritation and soreness, though the grubbiness of your child's face and neck is not a health risk whatever the neighbours might say.

Chemicals

These are not much help in dealing with wounds but a hypochlorite solution (such as Milton) can be used to kill bacteria on bottles, nappies and other baby equipment. Wash off milk from the bottles carefully first and remove solid matter from nappies (the solution can only sterilise something that is already reasonably free of bacteria-bearing matter). Read the instructions and ensure that the item to be sterilised is properly submerged and there are no air bubbles where bacteria can collect unharmed. The liquid should be changed daily and sterilised bottles and teats should be well rinsed. Wash your hands well before handling sterilised bottles or you will put the bacteria back in.

Heat kills bacteria

When you heat bacteria to boiling point you will kill them. However, new bacteria can return and start the process again unless you take care. Make sure your hands are clean before handling and store carefully (see below).

Bottles, dummies, and feeder cup lids carefully washed can then be sterilised by boiling in a pan with a lid, or by steaming. Nappies can also be sterilised by boiling or on the hottest cycle of some washing machines (check your instructions to make sure the water reaches boiling point).

Bacteria on food will also be killed by heat. If you are cooking, or reheating, animal products it is important to heat the food to boiling point all the way through. Be particularly careful about frozen meat or chicken which should be totally de-frosted before use and then cooked right through. Pre-cooked food which is then warmed up, but not properly heated through, is a major source of food poisoning.

If you give babies and toddlers food you have not cooked yourself you cannot be sure about the conditions in which it was prepared. Tinned or dried food or foods in jars are safe until they are opened, after which you have to treat them with the same care as any other food. If you use tins make sure your tin opener is regularly cleaned and not shared with the cat. Cooked foods from supermarkets 'deli' counters may well contain harmful bacteria. If you use them, be sure to follow cooking instructions very carefully.

Eggs have recently become a source of salmonella infection which is an absolute tragedy as they are an important source of iron and other nutrients and for many English children virtually the only fresh, whole food in their diet. The blame must fall squarely on egg producers who have been careless of hygiene, as well as the government which has allowed the profits of egg producers to come before the safety of our children. Anything made with raw egg, such as mayonnaise or home-made chocolate soufflé, is unsafe, and for children under a year it is best to avoid soft-boiled eggs, scrambled eggs or anything in which the egg is still runny. For older children the benefits of eating eggs probably outweigh the risk, so if they will only eat their eggs soft-boiled or scrambled you can probably risk it but still cook them on the hard side.

Ordinary tap water contains bacteria which may be too much for a young baby. In the first year it is wise to give only boiled water. You can keep it in a clean bottle in the fridge. Bottled milk (unless it has a green cap) has already been pasteurised or sterilised. You can give it to a six-month-old baby straight from the bottle but don't leave opened bottles hanging about. Put them straight back into the fridge. A part-consumed feed, or a jar which you have fed the baby from, should not be kept at all. Bacteria from the baby's mouth will now be in the food and already multiplying.

Cold stops bacteria developing

If food is frozen everything in it will also be frozen (including the bacteria). Cooked food should be cooled fast and put straight into the freezer for storage, otherwise bacteria can settle on it and start to multiply before freezing starts. Those bacteria will then start multiplying again as you warm up the food. That probably won't be a problem if you cook the food all the way through, but it is a risk worth avoiding.

If you are storing cooked food temporarily in a refrigerator you should cover it and put it straight into the fridge. Once in the fridge most bacteria do not thrive, so as long as you eat the food within a couple of days, there should be no danger. However, some bacteria (such as Listeria) can live in cold conditions, so if you have a young baby it is best to avoid using food which has been left in the fridge for more than a few hours.

Storage and preparation
Cooked and uncooked food must be handled separately. If the knife you used for cutting the chicken string is then used for salad carrots, the salmonella from the chicken may well end up, uncooked, inside your children. If you use this same board to cut raw meat and cheese you will cook the meat but some of the bacteria could end up in a cheese sandwich.

IF IN DOUBT THROW IT OUT is the best motto for food hygiene.

SAFETY

Keeping babies and young children safe is something we do almost instinctively. If a toddler darts out into a road every adult around will gasp and react immediately. Nevertheless accidents do happen and very often they are the result of lapses in our attention. Since we cannot keep our eyes glued on our kids all the time, and we don't want to keep them imprisoned in playpens, we need to a) find ways of making their environment as safe as possible, and b) make certain safety measures so habitual that we *never* forget them. This is the sort of accident which could be avoided by making safety routine:

> 'I had forgotten to strap her into the pushchair and, as we ran for the bus, I bumped the pushchair over a curb – she flew straight out on the road. Thank God there was no car coming so she only got a nasty grazed knee and banged head.'

If this is your first baby you will not yet have acquired the instinct for avoiding many of the hazards which are to come. It is worth trying to develop safety consciousness in advance so that you are not caught out. It is impossible to imagine that a tiny baby will soon be able to pull a hot cup of coffee off a table but it is worth trying to imagine it just in case she thinks of it first.

> 'The first time she learned to roll over she fell right off the bed. I simply hadn't thought about the possibility of her moving by herself.'

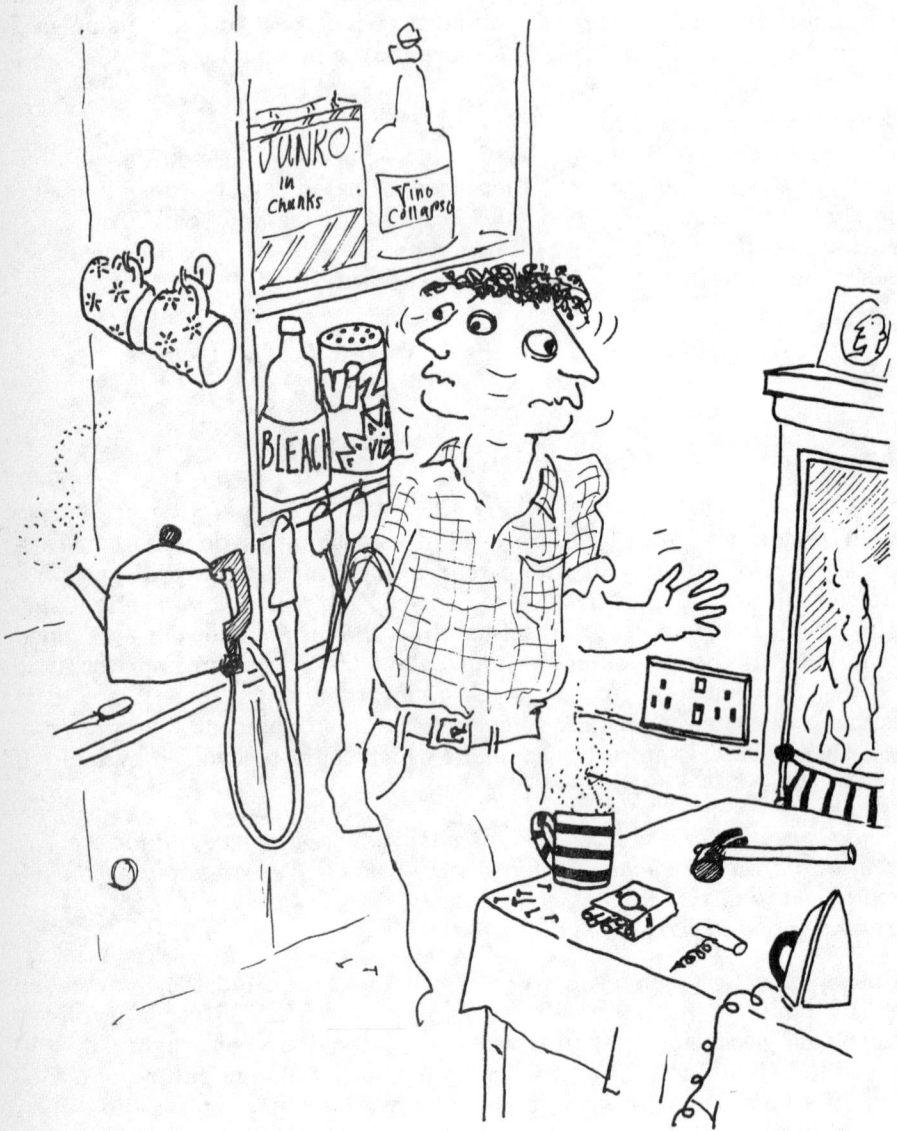

Home hazards

Look around your home or, better still, ask a friend with slightly older children to look for you. These are the sorts of hazards which should be dealt with now:

* Buy equipment with a British Standards Institute kite mark. This is particularly important if you are buying second-hand. Safety testing takes account of many hazards you wouldn't even have dreamed of.
* Do not give your baby a pillow to sleep on or leave her unattended in a quilted 'baby nest'. If the baby is not yet able to turn her head easily she could suffocate.
* Stairs are a hazard until your child can manage them easily. If you are a habitual door closer you may never leave your crawling baby unattended on the stairs. If not, you are safer with stair gates for the first eighteen months.
* All fires need guards which sit far enough away not to get too hot. Check that radiators are not hot enough to burn.
* Chemicals, medicines, cleaning fluids and alcohol should be kept well out of the way in a locked cabinet or high shelf. Make sure that your child cannot climb up to the shelf either. (I recently found my three-year-old standing on the basin and exploring the bathroom cabinet – she's a great climber!)
* Kettles, and their leads, should be kept well out of reach of all pre-school children.
* Get rid of coffee tables with sharp corners which are a hazard to crawlers and toddlers and make sure that tablecloths do not dangle invitingly where a newly standing baby can tug the whole lot (plus cups of hot tea) on to her head.
* Don't buy a baby walker. Your child will learn to walk quite happily without one and according to the child accident prevention trust they 'cause more accidents than any other single item of equipment'.
* Put furniture in front of electrical sockets or use socket covers to stop things being poked in.
* Check your windows. Upper floor windows should not open wide enough for a child to climb up and fall out. Can your landing windows and glass doors be fallen through? If they can, fit safety glass or replace with small-paned doors which are safe. Alternatively cover the glass with safety film, available at good chemists and babycare departments.
* Chest-type freezers can imprison a young child. Make sure your child is not able to lift the lid and climb in. Never throw fridges or freezers out without breaking door catches.
* Put all your own prized possessions out of reach so that you do not feel

compelled to wreak vengeance when your favourite record is fatally scratched.

* Provide older children with a safe space to store and play with their own toys.
* Treat small objects such as peanuts, marbles and pen tops as hazards. They can be swallowed, inhaled, and stuck into unlikely places. Keep them well out of reach of children under three.

Useful habits

* Never put hot water in the bath first. An adventurous child could climb into scalding water.
* Never leave a baby unattended on a high surface, in a high chair or in a bath, even if she is strapped in. Babies twist and fall when you least expect it and getting caught in the straps may be more dangerous than falling on the floor. Never strap a child into bed, for the same reason.
* Always put hot drinks in the middle of the table and well away from young children.
* Always check that children's food or drink is not hot enough to burn, before you put it on the table. A child can take a mouthful without stopping to check.
* Train yourself never to leave saucepans with their handles sticking out.
* Never leave a hot iron unattended and make sure that the flex is well wrapped round the iron when it is stored.
* Start putting the chain on the front door before your two-year-old learns how to open it and wanders into the street.
* Never allow a child to travel in a car or push chair without being strapped in.
* Teach three-year-olds how to use scissors and knives safely and make sure that sharp implements are always put away so that younger children cannot get at them.
* Make sure children don't wander round with things in their mouths (including food). They could choke if they fall.
* Teach children to take care of their own possessions and keep them away from younger siblings. Concern that their own things may be spoiled may help them to remember that their toys can also be a danger to a young child.
* Teach your children to swim but still don't leave them unattended near water. A young child can drown in a couple of inches. A paddling pool or even a bucket of water can be hazardous to a toddler. Even a child who has learned to swim may panic and inhale water if he falls into a swimming pool. Don't let your children use inflatable or swimming rings on a large stretch of water. They can be carried away by tide or winds.

* Be conscious that people who do not have children the same age as yours will have forgotten about the specific safety measures necessary. Get used to making a quick survey for hazards as soon as you arrive in an unfamiliar place. This is particularly important if you are leaving your child there.

Talking about safety

Under-threes find it very difficult to understand that their actions can have dangerous consequences. They may be intimidated into safety-consciousness but it is likely to be your anger, rather than the danger, that they fear. A four-year-old may understand that a street which is empty now could have a car on it in a minute but he will often forget in the heat of the moment.

Until children can both understand and remember safety rules, they need close attention, but it is never too soon to start teaching safety habits. Make sure that every time you cross a road you 'stop, look, listen and think' before crossing. If your three-year-old runs ahead towards a road crossing always *remind* her to stop before the corner. When you have to carry a knife or scissors point out that you only carry them with the blade pointing down. Never let your children climb on windowsills or balcony walls, even if you are holding them, and stop adults doing it in front of them.

It is best not to let under-fives play on the pavements at all if you can avoid it. It that is the only place a four-year-old can play, make clear rules, explain that you are making them because the pavements are dangerous, not because you want to spoil their fun, and be pretty fierce about them. Stay where you can hear them play and see them easily through a window. Make sure they know that they must come in as soon as the other children go home. Don't allow them to go into anyone else's house or flat without telling you.

Say exactly where they are allowed to go: 'no further than that tree and not past the blue van and if I see you step over the pavement on to the street you won't be allowed out for a week!' Look out of the window often so that they know you are watching and, ask responsible older children to keep an eye on them.

Stranger danger

Children are far more likely to be abused by people they know than by perfect strangers. Nevertheless we regularly read stories in the press about child abductions. It is hard to know how to keep a balance between frightening our children and keeping them safe. My own feeling is that, in both private situations and public ones, a child's personal confidence is her own best defence. A child who is frightened of adults is more likely to obey a stranger than a child who has a sense of her own rights as an individual.

If we always encourage our children to complain if they feel they are being unfairly treated, and we take their complaints seriously, they are a lot less likely to conceal abusing behaviour by other adults. If we dismiss our child's fears when he says he doesn't like a babysitter or child carer we are eroding his confidence in us as protectors. There is a very big difference between not liking to be left and not liking to be left with a particular person.

If we treat our children's bodies with respect, right from the start, they will learn that their bodies are their own and reject approaches that they have not initiated and do not want. If we let friends and relations plant kisses, without asking permission first, we are telling our children that they do not have control over who touches them. Children like to be cuddled and touched but they should be allowed to make the approach themselves to people they care for. They should not be made to feel that they are objects for the gratification of others. A girl who grows up feeling that she *owns* her own body is surely less likely to be misused than a girl who is brought up simply to fear men.

Children who feel confident with themselves and confident about our protection will be more able to deal confidently if dangerous situations do occur. We can also teach them how to stay safe:

* If you take your child into a crowded place consider writing his name and phone number on his arm.
* Say that if you get separated, your child should *not* look for you but stand still and wait to be found. It will be easier for you to find him than for him to find you.
* Teach your child her address as soon as she is able to repeat it to you.
* If your children get lost tell them only to get help from people accompanied by other children, or uniformed people in shops, police stations, railway stations, etc. Tell them never to get in a car.
* They should never go off with any adult (even someone they know) without telling you first.
* If a stranger tries to take them away they should make a lot of noise and kick his legs very hard indeed.

WHEN TO CALL A DOCTOR

ACCIDENTS

This book can give only the most basic guidelines. In an emergency you will not want to stop and look things up in any book. It is far better to be prepared by doing a basic First Aid course which will teach you how to do mouth-to-mouth respiration and deal confidently with accidents. It is also worthwhile investing in a First Aid book which will provide more detailed information.

Most accidents will be relatively trivial and require little more than reassurance from you. If *you* are worried, then *you* need reassurance and should turn to a professional for advice. That is what they are there for. It is best to get your child straight to an Accident and Emergency Unit where facilities such as X-ray equipment are available and tests can be done to ensure that there are no internal injuries. If there is no A and E department close by call your doctor for advice.

However anxious you are normally you will probably find that an icy calm comes over you if something happens to your child. It is as though someone else had taken over the controls. You can act calmly and rationally and you can keep your child calm and comfortable, nevertheless you are also in a shocked state. Try to avoid driving if you can. Take a friend with you to hospital if at all possible. Expect to collapse in a heap when it's all over and accept offers of help and comfort – you will need them.

In all cases avoid giving your child anything to eat or drink until you are sure that no real harm has been done. If an anaesthetic is necessary your child is safer with an empty stomach.

Concussion and head injuries

Call an ambulance immediately if a child is unconscious. While waiting, turn her carefully into the recovery position, making sure that her tongue is clear of her throat and not obstructing breathing. If you suspect that bones in the back may be broken, do not move the child at all – wait for the professionals.

If your child has been unconscious, even momentarily, take her to hospital for an X-ray to check for internal injury even if she appears to recover quickly.

After any bang on the head, pay attention to how your child behaves. If an egg-shaped bump appears or the wound is bleeding do not panic. Head wounds tend to look awful even when they are nothing to worry about. (See below for treating cuts.) After about twenty minutes she should be feeling better. If she still complains of blurred vision, dizziness, looks gray and pale or is breathing strangely consult your doctor or go straight to a hospital.

She may want to sleep. That is a normal reaction, but keep an eye on her and wake her occasionally. If you suspect she is lapsing into unconsciousness, call your doctor.

If the child is not breathing

You need to start mouth-to-mouth resuscitation. Make sure the tongue is not obstructing the air passages and clear any other obstructions you can

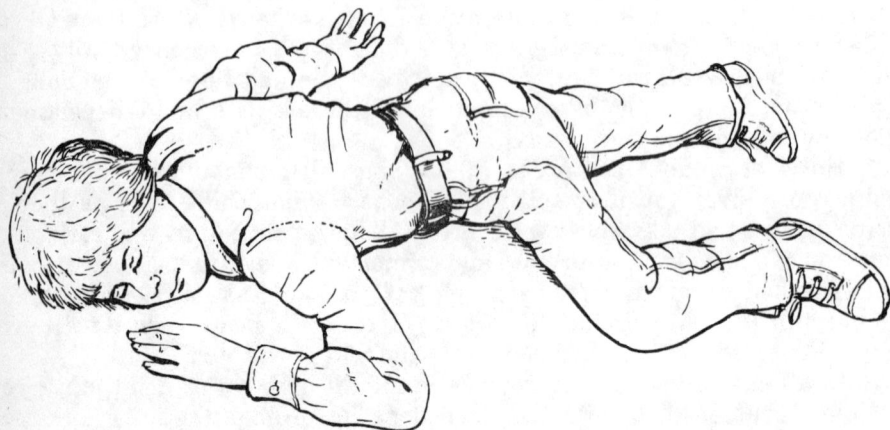

The recovery position

see. Put your hand under the chin, raising it slightly, so that the airways are as clear as possible. Put your mouth over the child's nose and mouth (hold the nose if you cannot manage this) and breath gently and rhythmically into his mouth. Stop when you see the chest rise, and start again when it deflates. If breathing resumes, put the child into the recovery position and get help as fast as you can.

If you suspect broken bones

If you think bones may be broken in the hip, thigh, back or neck, but the child is unconscious, try to keep her calm, and still, and call an ambulance. For other bones it may be easier for you to take your child to the hospital yourself if you have transport.

Cuts and abrasions

These provide direct entry for bacteria into the bloodstream. All young children get scratched and grazed as soon as they start to move so it is fortunate that our blood is quite good at defending itself. The best way to treat a cut or graze is to wash it under running water so that superficial dirt is removed. Slight bleeding is a good thing because the bacteria come out with the blood. Then just leave it to dry – the body will do the rest. If the child wants to dig in the garden or play in the sand, cover the wound up with plaster but don't leave it on for long as it will interfere with healing.

If the bleeding doesn't stop immediately, hold the edges of the wound together, or press against it with a clean handkerchief or gauze pad. Within three minutes, blood clotting should have taken over. If the blood is literally pouring out, you need to apply direct pressure to hold it in. A rolled up sock held, or tied, against the wound will probably work, or at least slow the flow. Tie it firmly against the wound while you decide what to do next.

See a doctor:
* If the blood is literally pouring out of a severed artery or the bleeding does not stop within minutes. Apply pressure (as above) and get to a hospital as fast as possible.
* If the wound is dirty, in which case you may need professional help to clean it up.
* If it is big, or deep enough, to need stitching to help it heal neatly and avoid scarring. This is particularly important for face wounds.
* If there is anything in the wound such as glass.
* If the area becomes red, hot and tender around the edges of the wound, or pus appears.

Burns

If the child is on fire, get her on to the ground and smother the flames with a blanket or coat or something similar. Then remove any clothing over the area and cool it down under cold running water. Burning may have penetrated beneath the surface of the skin and can do extensive damage. A burn which is the size of a saucer or more is potentially dangerous. Cover with a very clean cloth (perhaps a clean pillowcase) and go straight to the hospital. Smaller scalds should be covered with a loose gauze bandage to protect the area but don't put *anything* on it which could get stuck to the wound. Never use cream or any other medication. If you are unsure about the extent of scalding, see a doctor.

Animal bites

These should be seen by a doctor as bacteria from the animals teeth will have been introduced through the punctures.

Stings

These are painful but the pain usually goes away after about half an hour. However if the child is allergic to the sting or there are a large number of them she may go into shock. Signs would be that the child is generally unwell, short of breath and dazed. This is an emergency. Call an ambulance or take her straight to the nearest hospital.

Foreign bodies

Anything in ears, nose, vagina etc. should only be removed if you can get at them very easily and are certain that you will not push the object further in. If in doubt contact your doctor or go to the hospital.

Poisons

Any poison swallowed should be dealt with immediately in most cases by getting the child to vomit. If you are not sure what the substance is or how much the child has swallowed, get the container and the child to the nearest hospital as fast as possible. If you have easy access to a phone, and you are not sure whether the substance is harmful, call your doctor first for advice.

Choking

If your child chokes on an object or lump of food he will probably cough it out again. If he is unable to cough, or his breathing is obstructed, hold him upside-down, or over your knee with his head hanging well down below his body, and thump him firmly between the shoulder blades several times. If that doesn't work and breathing is affected, do mouth-to-mouth respiration, in between attempts to dislodge the object and get help fast, if necessary, by opening a window and yelling for help.

An electric shock

This may throw the child across the room and away from the source of electricity. If it does not, do not touch the child yourself or you will also get a shock. First turn off the supply or, failing that, use a broom or chair to push the child away from it. If the child is not breathing do mouth-to-mouth resuscitation (as above), turn him to the recovery position (see diagram) and get help immediately.

ILLNESS

Most of us learn very quickly to spot signs of illness in a child. We may not know what is wrong but we can tell when something is 'not normal'. The hard part is being able to work out whether the 'not normal' means ill, or just different. Or, if the child clearly is ill, whether the illness is *potentially* serious, or will clear up by itself.

'It's 10 pm and my baby is running a temperature. I feel perfectly able
to cope now but I know that if she wakes at 2 am I will feel very anxious.
Should I call a doctor now, knowing that the answer will be, "Give her

some Calpol and see how she is in the morning," or should I wait and see, running the risk of a late-night phone-call instead?'

Making judgements about a child's health is very much a learning process. We begin at the very beginning with our first baby, and as the child gets older or we have one or two more, our expertise gradually increases. We start to learn when we can safely treat illness ourselves and when we need to see a doctor. As we are learning we need help. Each time we ask advice from a doctor, health visitor, or even more experienced parent, we are adding to the sum of our knowledge. A caring doctor or health visitor should understand this and be prepared to give advice whenever *we* need it. Even those of us who know a lot about medicine may find it hard to make clear judgements about our own children. We all need support and advice from time to time.

If your child seems ill, the evening approaches, and you want advice and reassurance, you should not feel embarrassed or guilty about asking for

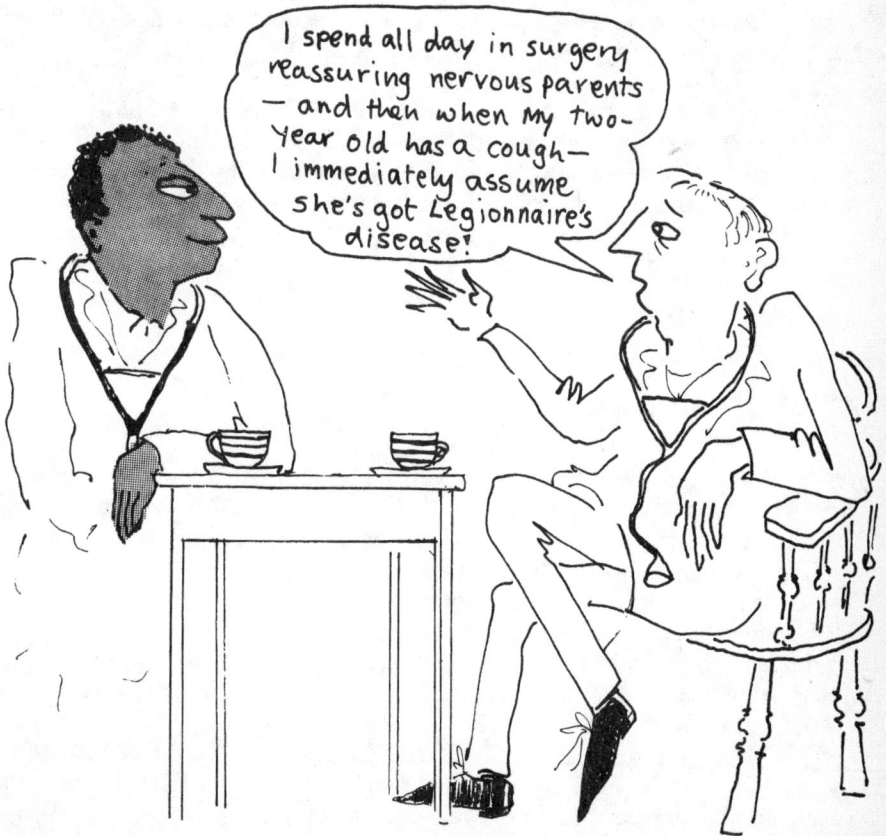

it. You will save yourself a lot of anxiety if you make that call and talk to someone about your child earlier rather than later. The advice may well be to see how things are in the morning but you will feel a great deal better if you have *shared* your anxiety. If you feel calmer, you will cope more calmly with whatever the night brings. In some cases the doctor may choose to visit earlier and make an assessment rather than risk being woken in the early hours of the morning.

During the day it always seems easier to make decisions. If you decide that medical attention is necessary you need to consider whether you would be better off taking the child to the doctor, or whether you need the doctor to come to you. It is usually quicker to wrap the child up and take her to the doctor, even if she seems to be seriously ill. If you don't have a car, your child is too big to carry or to take in a pram or buggy, or you feel that a journey to the doctor will make your child sicker, then ask the doctor to come to you. This will usually take a lot longer because the doctor has many other commitments. If it is an emergency say so. You may be advised to call an ambulance rather than wait. If you suspect that the illness is contagious (for example she is covered in spots), warn the receptionist. The doctor will probably want to keep you well away from other people.

If you are feeling very worried about your child you may desperately want your doctor to *do* something. Sometimes that will be what your child needs. More often, the most useful thing your doctor can give you is the confidence to carry on nursing your child yourself. A healthy child can, in most cases, deal pretty well with passing viruses and bacteria. In fact the experience of getting ill, and getting over it, is part of the process of building resistance to disease. You do not need the help of medication unless your child is facing a disease which he cannot fight off without help.

WHEN IS ILLNESS SERIOUS?

If your child seems ill she probably *is* ill. The things to look out for are a change from what is normal *for her*. A baby who just seems floppy and listless may be a lot iller than one who has a roaring temperature. If a child who normally has a healthy appetite suddenly refuses to eat, keep an eye on her. If your bouncy three-year-old becomes quiet and grizzly there may well be something on the way. If a toddler with a temperature otherwise seems quite well take steps to lower the temperature, but don't worry unduly. If, on the other hand, she has a low temperature in addition to seeming very listless and low, you should probably see a doctor.

IF THIS IS YOUR FIRST BABY REMEMBER THAT IT IS ALL RIGHT TO ASK FOR ADVICE WHENEVER YOU ARE WORRIED. People may chuckle about over-anxious first-time parents, but they know that illness can move very fast in a small baby and it is better to be over-anxious than under-anxious.

EMERGENCY CHECKLIST

Get urgent help:
 * If the baby has a fit or convulsion, or turns blue or very pale.
 * If breathing is very quick, comes in grunts and seems difficult.
 * If the baby seems unusually drowsy or unresponsive or exceptionally hard to wake.

Get medical advice:
 * If your baby seems unusually hot, cold or floppy.
 * If the baby vomits frequently or doesn't feed or has frequent watery stools. All three symptoms together need urgent attention.
 * For a hoarse cough or noisy breathing.
 * For crying which is unusual or unusually prolonged.

If you are worried about your baby's health get advice from your doctor whatever the time of day. If after seeing the doctor, the condition does not start to improve rapidly, contact him or her again the same day.

Diarrhoea and Vomiting

Some babies and children vomit for no obvious reason and a couple of bouts of diarrhoea may just be a reaction to a change in diet. Avoid giving the child anything to eat, but give as much liquid as you can get into her. It is important to keep the liquid level high because the major danger is from dehydration. Avoid all milk (including formula) except breast milk (which you should always continue). Plain boiled water or well diluted fruit juice is fine. The best drink of all, particularly for a baby, is an electrolyte solution which may be prescribed by a doctor. You can make it up yourself by adding a level tablespoon of sugar, plus a pinch of salt, to a pint of boiled water and then cooling it in the fridge.

If, the child seems to be well by the next meal time, re-introduce bottle formula, if you use it, but dilute by about half as much again. For children on solids try any of the following (recommended by a naturopath): lightly stewed apple (which contains pectin); live yoghurt (which contains lactobacillus or acidophillus, both of which help the child's natural defences against bacteria); or plain boiled rice. If the child throws all this straight up (or out), be more insistent about avoiding all solids for a few hours longer.

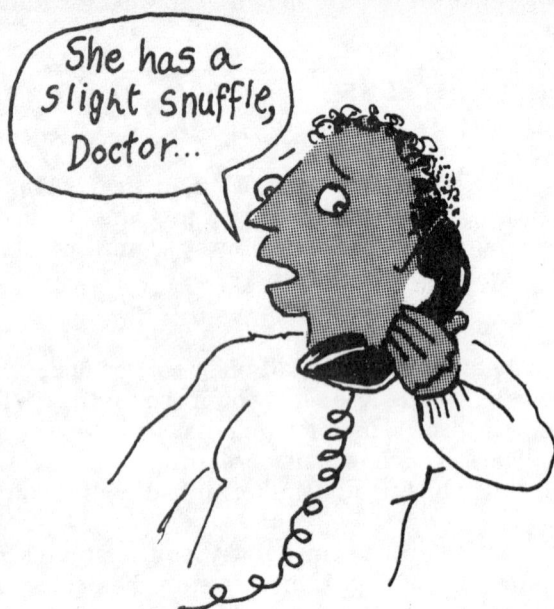

She has a slight snuffle, Doctor...

Call a doctor

* If a child below a year old has diarrhoea *and* vomiting. This is potentially dangerous. Encourage your baby to drink, and contact a doctor within four hours. If the baby also has a temperature don't wait – get straight to a doctor or hospital.

* If a baby has diarrhoea alone make an appointment to see a doctor, but in the meantime make sure she is getting plenty to drink (see above). If the condition has cleared before you get there, so much the better. Get urgent medical attention if: the baby does not want to drink; is drinking plenty but seems floppy, pale and sunken-eyed; seems to be taking in less liquid than is going out.

* Older children are not so vulnerable but you should still see a doctor if *you* feel concerned about your child's general wellbeing; if the vomiting is frequent, or lasts more than a day; if the child is in pain or is passing blood; if the child seems particularly dozy and the skin looks grey and lifeless.

* In all cases, if you have seen a doctor and been given advice or medication and the condition does not respond quickly, contact her again. A condition which may seem trivial after the first twelve hours will be serious if it does not come under pretty speedy control. The same rules apply – if your child seems ill, listless, greyish, and is not taking in more liquid than he is losing he is still in a dangerous condition even if he did see the doctor yesterday or the day before. It may be necessary

to test for a bacterial infection or even to admit into hospital for rehy-
dration. Ask your doctor if she wants you to bring a sample in with you.
* Persistent bouts of diarrhoea could be a sign of food intolerance, allergy,
  or some other problem. If simple remedies do not bring the condition
  under control ask for a referral to a paediatrician.

Temperatures

In most cases a temperature is not much to worry about. Young children
often run a temperature for little apparent reason and usually they will
have disappeared by the next day. However, it can be a sign of underlying
infection, and in some children a temperature can spiral very high, very
fast, causing febrile convulsions (see below).

There is usually no need to take your child's temperature. You can see
it: her body will be hot to the touch and you will probably notice a feverish
brightness in her eyes. If it seems very high you may want to find out exactly
what it is in order to tell the doctor. If your child seems under the weather,
but you are not quite sure what action to take, taking her temperature will
provide additional information.

In all cases, if a child seems feverish, cool her down by removing bed-
clothes and clothing, and fanning or sponging her with tepid water. This
may be enough to get the temperature under control. If it doesn't start to
fall immediately, give her a paracetamol suspension such as Calpol, and
continue the cooling process while you wait for it to take effect. If the child
feels very shivery and sensitive you may not be able to sponge her without
causing real distress. Give the paracetamol straight away and then start to
cool her down as soon as the shivering subsides.

Stay with her until you are sure that her temperature is dropping. She
may well want to sleep. Make sure she is wearing as little clothing as
possible so that heat is not trapped against her skin. This is particularly
important for a young baby. Encourage her to drink when she wakes to
avoid dehydration.

Call a doctor
* If the temperature continues to rise and fall for more than twenty-four
  hours.
* If there are additional symptoms such as pain or vomiting, or the child
  seems particularly unwell.
* If the combination of paracetamol and cooling is not bringing her temperature under control.
* If the temperature continues to rise uncontrollably. In about 3 per cent
  of children this could result in febrile convulsions.

Febrile convulsions

These are most likely to happen at the start of a fever if the temperature rises very fast. The child's body will go rigid and then jerk uncontrollably. A fit rarely lasts more than a couple of minutes. Stay with the child to make sure that she doesn't hurt herself but do nothing to intervene. As soon as the fit is over, contact a doctor. If the fit has not subsided within 3 minutes phone or call for help.

If you have access to a car and someone to drive you, it may be better to take the child straight to a hospital rather than wait for a doctor to come. In most cases the fit will be over, and the child asleep, by the time you get to a doctor. Your child may be admitted overnight for observation, or your doctor may judge that this is not necessary. This depends as much on the doctor's individual practice as on your child's condition so don't be unduly alarmed if admission is recommended.

Coughs and colds

Many babies get their first cold very early, particularly if they have older brothers or sisters. In most cases it will result in no more than a blocked nose. With a baby this can also cause feeding problems because it is hard to suck and breathe at the same time. In this case you can ask your doctor about decongestant nose drops. It may help to put a pillow *under* the baby's mattress as she sleeps, so that her head is higher than her body, which may prevent her nose blocking and waking her up all night. Older children may also prefer to sleep with a pillow during a cold.

In most cases a snotty nose and cough (a necessary reaction to keep mucous away from the chest and lungs) is a familiar and passing matter which is really not worth worrying about. Don't be too concerned either about the horrible hacking and croaking which you may hear when your child wakes up. He has collected mucous all through the night and is now getting rid of it. In a couple of hours he will probably sound less alarming. Some children also throw up whenever they have a cold – this is just a rather less pleasant way of getting rid of the mucous collecting in their stomachs.

Children are usually more comfortable (particularly at bed time) if you allow them to breathe in plenty of damp, steamy air. A bath may be enough to create the right conditions, or sit your child in the kitchen, close the door, and put on a couple of pans of water to boil while you read a bedtime story.

Do not give cold cures to a child. They will not cure and may be danger-ous. You might like to consider a naturopathic approach, and cut out milk products when your child has a cold. This may keep down the amount of mucous produced.

When to see a doctor

A cold is caused by a virus for which there is no known cure, so there is very little point in seeing a doctor unless you feel that there may be a *secondary* infection in addition to a cold.

* Runny eyes and pain in the ears should be investigated. A *bacterial* infection may have set up home in the mucous created by the virus, in which case you *may* need antibiotic treatment.

* A child who gets worse rather than better after the first twenty-four hours may have some additional problem which should be investigated.

* Wheezy, laboured breathing, particularly if it seems very fast, may indicate a chest infection or possibly asthma. It is not the amount of noise produced which matters but whether or not there is any effect on the child's breathing. If you are not sure, see your doctor. She can listen to the child's chest and advise you whether there appears to be any infection and what, if anything, you should do about it. If your child is clearly struggling for breath, contact your doctor immediately, night or day.

* Asthma is a recurring condition. If your child has asthma you will need advice on prevention as well as medication for controlling the condition.

* A loud, barking cough, possibly combined with wheezing, may well be croup. Your child will probably wake terrified and apparently unable to breathe. You may well feel just as terrified. Your first action must be to calm your child, so you will have to push your fear away and cope with it later. He will breathe more easily if he is calm. Then get as much steam in the room as possible. The simplest solution is to take the child into the bathroom and turn on the hot taps, or into the kitchen while you boil pans of water. If there is someone else around, get them to call a doctor. If not, wait until the child's breathing eases and call the doctor yourself. Don't leave the child alone with boiling pans. If you have to go out to phone the doctor, take the child with you. The cold air will help his breathing.

With the first attack of croup you should call a doctor. It is not likely to be dangerous but in rare cases it is, so you must make sure. Since croup is a recurring condition, ask the doctor's advice about how to cope with later attacks. You will certainly feel a great deal less frightened the second time round and better able to make a judgement. A child with severe croup should not be left alone. Take him into your bed, or sleep in his room, and invest in a kettle which does not switch itself off when it boils so that you can easily get steam into the atmosphere. (Make sure you don't fall asleep with it on as you could start a fire.)

Rashes

Spots and blotches make frequent appearances in children. Tiny raised spots with watery heads may be simply a heat rash. Check that you are not over-wrapping your baby (see p. 184). A rash may be the early warning signs of allergy (see p. 125). If a rash appears within hours of trying a new food, try it again in a couple of weeks and see if you get a reaction (in which case avoid that food for the time being). Patches of raised, rough, red skin may be the start of eczema, which is itself nearly always allergic in origin though it is not often easy to pinpoint what is causing it.

Redness around the vagina or nappy area may be straightforward nappy rash or thrush (both of these are discussed on p. 136). However the most common reason is a virus. Many virus rashes come and go overnight without any other ill effect. Other are associated with well-known childhood diseases such as chickenpox, measles or rubella.

If your child is spotty but otherwise well, try to keep her away from crowded places where she may be in contact with pregnant women. A virus which barely affects a healthy child can damage a developing foetus. Nurseries usually have a clear policy about dealing with childhood diseases and may insist on lengthy exclusions to keep the infection from spreading. Child-minders vary in their approach. Many of them take the view that children may as well get these diseases while they are young and will take your child (infectious or not) provided she is reasonably cheerful.

An eczema or allergy rash will not cause illness as such but it may make your child very miserable. Eczema often starts on the cheeks. If you are lucky it will stay there or only appear in a few places and cause little real difficulty. It may however spread. The itching will in turn cause your child to scratch which will lead to inflammation and pain. An unhappy baby usually means unhappy parents. Your child may wake often in the night, miserable with the feeling of her own skin, and be hard to settle by day.

There are a few basic tips which will help all eczema sufferers: keep clothing as light as possible and avoid synthetic materials which do not 'breathe'. Cotton vests and tee shirts and loose cotton trousers will keep the affected areas covered (and less vulnerable) and allow air to circulate. Avoid soaps and bubble baths – your doctor can prescribe aqueous cream for use in the bath and on the skin.

When to see a doctor
  * If your child is ill as well as spotty, ring your doctor for advice. He or she may prefer to visit rather than spread the virus to other patients in the waiting room. Even if she is not very ill, you may also want a clear diagnosis so that you know which diseases your child has had (and is therefore immune to) and just how long she is likely to be infectious.
  * If you suspect that your child has eczema take her to the doctor. This

condition cannot be cured but it is as well to have good advice about how to cope with something which may recur frequently and cause a lot of discomfort. There are creams which can be used to relieve the condition and some contain cortico steroids. They are effective but should be used with extreme caution as they are absorbed into the skin and tend to lower the child's general resistance to infection. Your doctor may prescribe an antihistamine solution to give your baby at night. This should relieve the itching and make your child sleepy. However children vary in their reaction to antihistamines. It can occasionally cause them to be more wakeful than ever! As with all medications, these should be used sparingly and kept for those times when you all really need them.

* This condition may be best treated homoeopathically (see 'Help' for the addresses). If it is severe, you may want to try (with medical help) an elimination diet which could help you to trace the foods which are causing the problems (see Allergies, p. 121).

Eyes and ears

Eye infections are quite common in babies and young children. If an eye seems red and a bit sticky, try self-help treatment first. Add a little salt to some freshly boiled, cooled water, and use cotton wool to wipe the stickiness away from the eyelid. Do this several times a day. If the condition hasn't cleared in twenty-four hours, see a doctor. You may need antibiotic drops or cream. It may be very hard to get the drops or cream into the eye, and unless the antibiotic goes to the right place it will do no good. If your child is a deep sleeper you could try applying it when she is asleep.

Ear infections can be the bane of a baby's life. There may be absolutely nothing to indicate what the problem is but you will almost certainly know that something is wrong because your baby will be in pain and crying. Often, but not always, the infection will be accompanied by a temperature and may be triggered by a cold. If you call a doctor for unexplained crying she should always check your baby's ears for signs of infection.

Once you have had the first infection diagnosed you will quite quickly become expert at diagnosing another one. Don't wait to get medical help (day or night). The sooner your baby is on antibiotics, the sooner the pain will go away. You may however want to talk to your doctor or an alternative practitioner (naturopath or homoeopath) about ways of avoiding recurring infections if at all possible. As a first step it is important to use earplugs in the bath and the swimming pool and keep the ears dry. Never, ever, attempt to clean the inside of a child's ears or put anything else inside them.

If your child has a history of recurring ear infections you should ask for tests (see p. 38) to find out whether his hearing has been affected. When your child is about two, you may be asked to consider the insertion of grommets – tiny plastic or metal implants which help the ear to drain more efficiently. These can be dramatically effective initially, but the improvement does not always last. You should discuss this with your doctor.

GENERAL ADVICE AND CHECK-UPS

Midwives

They are experts in the care of babies in the first ten days of life. You should be visited regularly by your midwife for the first ten days after you get home. She should give you a phone number to contact her if you need help in between calls. Before she leaves you she should provide information about baby clinics and health visitors.

Health visitors

They are supposed to visit all new mothers just to see how you are managing and whether you need any advice. Since they have very big case loads they may just pop in once, decide that you are doing fine, and move on. If you do not feel that you are doing fine you can ring and ask her to see you. Health visitors can be wonderful (and some can be worse than useless). They can provide a shoulder to cry on if you are at the end of your tether as well as practical advice on teething and tantrums. Some now run groups for new parents, either around a particular issue (such as sleep problems) or as a postnatal group. Health visitors also run baby clinics (see below).

General practitioners

They have a very special rôle for new parents. A good GP will make you feel happy about asking questions even if, in retrospect, you can see that you were getting things completely out of proportion. If your GP does not give you this feeling of confidence you may want to consider finding another. Of course anyone has a right to feel irritated if they are called at 11 pm because Johnny has a cold, but there is nothing worse than being alone with a sick child and feeling unable to 'bother the doctor'. You may well find that a doctor who has herself been through the anxiety of new parenthood will be particularly reassuring.

Well baby clinics

These provide exactly what they suggest: a service for well babies. They will not give you advice if your baby is ill and they cannot prescribe medicines (unless the clinic is run by your own doctor). The service is mainly aimed at checking whether your baby is developing at a rate within the normal range. If he is not, they can do a basic assessment of the problem and pass you on to specialists. The checking usually involves weighing and measuring, basic developmental tests and hearing and sight tests. Immunisations are also done at this clinic.

For a first baby this service may be a useful way of learning more about your child, and a back-up for your own parenting. Once you have had the experience of one child you may decide to use the clinic only for innoculation. However, it is still worth checking with a clinic if you are at all worried about your baby's progress.

HELP

ORGANISATIONS

Postnatal and parent support
Association for Postnatal Illness, 7 Gowan Avenue, London SW6 (01–731 4867). Advice for mothers with severe postnatal depression.

Cry-sis, BM Cry-sis, London WC1N 3XX (01–404 5011). For parents of crying babies. Phone for local phone number.

Disabled Parents Contact Register, c/o the National Childbirth Trust (see below.) Advice and contact for parents with disabilities.

Foundation for the Study of Infant Deaths, 15 Belgrave Square, London SW1X 8PS. Support for parents who have experienced a cot death.

Gingerbread, 25 Wellington Street, London WC2E 7BN (01–240 0953/4). Self-help organisation for single parents, branches nationwide.

MAMA, 5 Westbury Gardens, Luton, Beds (0582 422253). Countrywide local groups for new mothers, some providing special help for those suffering from postnatal depression.

National Childbirth Trust, Alexandra House, Oldham Terrace, Acton, London W3 (01–992 8637).

The Parent Network, 44–46 Caversham Road, London NW5 2DS (01–485 8535). Trained leaders run parents groups to discuss family relationships and develop strategies.

Women's Therapy Centre, 6–9 Manor Gardens, London N7 (01–263 6200).

Parents in crisis
OPUS, 106 Godstone Road, Whyteleafe, Croydon CR3 0EB (01–645 0496). Support groups and day centres for families under stress.

Parents Anonymous, 6–9 Manor Gardens, London N7 6LA (nightline 01–669 8900). For parents at the end of their tether who fear they could hurt their children.

Premature babies
Bliss-Link, 44/45 Museum Street, London WC1 (01–831 9393). Support group for parents of babies in special care.

Nippers, 49 Allison Road, Acton, London W3. (Parents' support group).

Scottish Premature Babies Support Group, 5 Boghead Road, Lenzie, Glasgow.

Twins and Multiple Births Association, 54 Windmill Drive, Croxley Green, Rickmansworth, Herts WD3 3FE.

Breastfeeding support
Association of Breastfeeding Mothers, 10 Herschell Road, London SE23 1EN (01–778 4769). This is a 24-hour advice line with telephone numbers across the UK.

La Lêche League, BM 3424 (01–404 5011 daytime). Has local groups all over the country.

National Childbirth Trust, Alexandra House, Oldham Terrace, Acton, London W3 (01–992 8637). Has breastfeeding counsellors who will give telephone and personal advice.

Allergies
Asthma Research Council and Asthma Society, 300 Upper Street, London N1 (01–226 2269).

National Eczema Society, Tavistock House, North Tavistock Square, London WC1H 9SR (01–388 4097).

Hyperactive Children's Support Group, Mrs Sally Bunday, 59 Meadowside, Angmering, West Sussex BN16 4BW. Provides information on hyperactivity and allergy.

Homoeopathy is available on the NHS from:
Bristol Homoeopathic Hospital, Cotham Road, Cotham, Bristol BS6 6JU (0272 33068).

Glasgow Homoeopathic Hospital, 1000 Great Western Road, Glasgow G12 0NR (041–339 0382).

Liverpool The Mossley Hill Hospital, Park Avenue, Liverpool L18 8BU (051–724 3355).

London Royal London Homoeopathic Hospital, 60 Great Ormond Street, London WC1N 3HR (01–837 3091).

Tunbridge Wells Homoeopathic Hospital, Church Road, Tunbridge Wells, Kent TN1 1JU (0892 42977).

Naturopaths can be contacted through *The British Naturopathic and Osteo-pathic Association*, Frazer House, 6 Netherhall Gardens, London NW3 5RR (01–435 7320).

Children with disabilities
In Touch, 10 Norman Road, Sale, Cheshire. M33 3DF (061–962 4441). Contacts and support for parents of children with lesser known disabilities.

Voluntary Council for Handicapped Children, National Children's Bureau, 8 Wakeley Street, London EC1V 7QE (01–278 9441). For information about organisations dealing with disabilities.

Children in hospital
I Can, Invalid Children's Aid Nationwide, 198 City Road, London EC1V 2JH (01–608 2462).

National Association for the Welfare of Children in Hospital, Argyle House, 29–31 Euston Road, London NW1 2SD (01–833 2041).

Bereaved parents
Compassionate Friends, 5 Lower Clifton Hill, Clifton, Bristol (0272 292778). Phone for a local number. Counselling and support nationwide.

Benefits, Employment Rights
Child Poverty Action Group, Welfare Rights Office, 4–5 Bath Street, London EC1V 9PY (01–253 3406).

Maternity Alliance, 15 Britannia Street, London WC1X 9JP (01–837 1265). Provides advice and publications about employment and welfare rights for new parents.

NCCL Rights for Women Unit, 21 Tabard Street, London SE1 4LA.

Child care
Childcare Now, c/o National Childcare Campaign, Wesley House, 4 Wild Court, London WC2B 5AU (01–045 5617). Campaign for high quality day care supported by all the major child care organisations.

National Childminding Association, 25 Wellington Row, London E2 7BB (01–464 6164).

National Out of School Alliance, Oxford House, Derbyshire Street, Bethnal Green Road, London E2 6HG. Campaigns nationally and locally for after-school and holiday care.

New Ways to Work, 309 Upper Street, London N1 2TX (01–226 4026). Runs a job-sharing register and will give advice about employment contracts for job sharers and negotiators.

Working Mothers Association, 77 Holloway Road, London N7 8JZ (01–700 5771). Has local support groups and campaigns for better employment rights and child care locally and nationally.

Workplace Nurseries, 77 Holloway Road, London N7 8JZ (01–700 0281). Campaigns for a change in the tax law to aid workplace nurseries, and provides an advisory service for employers and trades unions interested in setting up workplace nurseries.

Local help

If you are concerned about your child there is often help available locally. The phone numbers given above are mostly national numbers, but many of them can give you a local contact. These are the usual routes to local assistance:
    Your general practitioner can give you advice and referral for most things both medical and developmental. If you suspect that your child has an undiagnosed health problem or disability you can ask for referral to a *paediatrician* (a specialist in children). You may also be referred to a range of health care workers such as physiotherapists or audiologists. If the problem is about toilet training ask for referral to an *enuresis* clinic. For behavioural problems you can be referred to a *Child Guidance Clinic* and for hearing problems to an *audiologist*.

Health visitors may run special clinics or groups for parents of children with sleep problems, or general postnatal support groups. They are often a good source of advice about local groups and services of all kinds.

The Social Services department of your council should provide information about benefits and allowances and they have a list of local organisations dealing with specific handicapping conditions. Help and advice may be practical as well as supportive. This department also holds lists of registered child care facilities and drop-in centres.

Child Guidance Clinics can be approached directly for help with any problems you may be having with your child's behaviour.

The Educational Psychologist working with your local schools may be a useful source of advice, reassurance and help about developmental problems and will often see children before nursery age.

BOOKS

These books (and some articles) are divided in a fairly arbitrary way according to my use of them in the book. If you don't find what you are looking for in the obvious place, you may find it somewhere else. They are listed according to title, not author.

Parenting

Balancing Acts: on being a mother ed. Katherine Gieve (Virago, 1989). Powerful and moving descriptions of motherhood.

Dream Babies by Christian Hardyment (Cape, 1983). An antidote to child care guides.

From Here to Maternity by Ann Oakley (Pelican, 1981). Interviews with women during pregnancy and afterwards. A riveting read and a comforting insight into other people's lives.

Falling for Love by Sue Sharpe (Virago, 1987). Interviews with teenage mothers.

Fathering by Ross D. Parke (Fontana, 1981).

The Father Figure by Lorna McKee and Margaret O'Brian (Tavistock, 1982).

Getting Pregnant Our Way by Lisa Saffron (Women's Health Information Centre, 1986) Available from the WHRRIC, 52 Featherstone Street, London EC1Y 8RT. Women who have become pregnant using 'donor insemination' talk about the practical and emotional aspects.

Give and Take in Families edited by Julia Brannen and Gail Wilson (Allen and Unwin, 1987). Studies in resource allocation within the family (could have been subtitled 'Father Takes All!').

The New Our Bodies Ourselves edited by Angela Phillips and Jill Rakusen (Penguin, 1989).

Postnatal Depression by Vivienne Welburn (Fontana, 1980).

Rocking the Cradle by Gillian Hanscombe and Jackie Forster (Peter Owen, 1981). Interviews with lesbian mothers.

Why Children? edited by Stephanie Dowrick and Sibyl Grundberg (The Women's Press, 1980).

Child development

Baby Language by Marie Messenger Davies, Eva Lloyd and Andreas Scheffler (Unwin Hyman, 1987). On the development of language.

Creative Play by Dorothy Einon (Viking, 1985).

Developmental Psychology by David Shaffer (Brooks/Cole (Calif.), 1985).

How Children Fail by John Holt (Pelican, 1971). This book is about school-children but it is full of lessons which parents would do well to learn before their children start 'learning to fail'.

The Baby Massage Book by Tina Heinl (Coventure, 1983).

Toys and Playthings by John and Elizabeth Newson (Penguin, 1979).

Young Children Learning by Barbara Tizard and Martin Hughes (Fontana, 1984).

Children with disabilities
Children of Silence by Kathy Robinson (Gollancz, 1987). A moving account of a family coming to terms with deafness.

Parents and the Handicapped Child by Margaret Marshal (Julia Macrae, 1982). Practical help for parents.

Problem Solving
A Good Enough Parent by Bruno Bettelheim (Thames and Hudson, 1987). Words of wisdom, particularly useful for older children.

The Experience of Breastfeeding by Sheila Kitzinger (Penguin, 1979).

Breast is Best by Andrew and Penelope Stanway (Pan, 1983).

Crying Baby: how to cope by Pat Gray (Wisebuy, 1987). The author, herself the mother of a crying baby started Cry-sis, the help-line for parents (see organisations, above).

The Crying Baby by Sheila Kitzinger (Viking, 1989). Interviews with parents of persistently crying babies, a round-up of existing theory about crying, plus support and advice.

'Community Survey of children of one to two years with sleep disturbances' by Naomi Richman, unpublished paper, Great Ormond Street Hospital, 1982.

'Infant sleeping difficulties and subsequent development' by J. Golding and A. Fredrick. Report on Child Health and Education Study, 1970 National Cohort (*Health Visitor*, August 1986).

My Child Won't Sleep by Jo Douglas and Naomi Richman (Penguin, 1984). A practical guide for parents of children with sleep problems, based on many years of practical experience with families.

The Politics of Food by Geoffrey Cannon (Century, 1988).

'Food allergy and CNS in childhood' in *Food Allergy and Intolerance* by J. Brostoff and S. Challacombe (eds) (Balliere Tindall, 1987).

Prescription for Poor Health ed. Jean Conway (Maternity Alliance, 1988).

'Controlled trial of oligionatigenic treatment in hyperkinetic syndrome' by J. Eggar et al (*The Lancet*, 9 March, 1985).

Care sharing

The Care of Young Children by Barbara Tizard (Thomas Coram Research Unit, 1986). A booklet (£2.00) which sums up recent research on the effects of daycare on children.

Babies in Daycare edited by Veronica Williams (Daycare Trust, 1989). £4.95 from the National Childcare Campaign.

Day Care by Alison Clarke-Stewart (Fontana, 1982). An international perspective, a bit out of date now.

Double Identity by Sue Sharpe (Pelican, 1984). The lives of working women.

Employers Guide to Day Care by The Working Mothers Association, 1989. £8.50 by post from the Association (see organisations above, for address).

Fathers, Childbirth and Work by Colin Bell, Lorna McKee and Karren Priestley (Equal Opportunities Commission, 1983).

For the Children's Sake by Caroline New and Miriam David (Pelican, 1985). A socialist feminist analysis of children in society.

Inside Story by the Maternity Alliance, 1989. Women's experiences of returning to work after maternity leave with negotiating guidelines for improving employment rights.

Male and Female by Margaret Mead (Penguin, 1962). An anthropological investigation of gender roles.

Maternity Rights, the Experience of Working Women by W. W. Daniels (Policy Studies Institute, 1980). Still the only comprehensive study of what happens to women's jobs after pregnancy.

Mothering by Rudolph Schaffer (Fontana, 1977). A study of what mothering is (and isn't).

INDEX